LIFE
To The
FULLEST

by Dan Brannan

Printed in the United States of America

First Edition — May 1996

ISBN 0-9650228-1-1

Published by Dan Brannan Publications
P.O. Box 1708
Seneca, SC 29679

Printed by Faith Printing Co.
4210 Locust Hill Rd.
Taylors, SC 29687

Cover design by Bryan Lee and Dana Alder

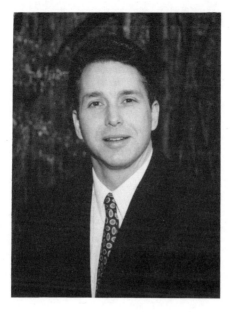

Imagine that your life is going about as well as you hoped; then, suddenly, a mysterious disease strikes, leaving you on the brink of death before you come roaring back from it.

That's what happened to Dan Brannan, a young, vibrant man who was on top of the world before diabetes struck down his dreams. But diabetes didn't kill his fighting spirit.

In this book, Dan, a newspaper editor in Seneca, S.C., tells his remarkable story and the stories of others who haven't let diabetes become a death sentence for them. A portion of the proceeds of this book will go for research into and treatment for diabetes.

Table of Contents

Introduction

I have known Dan Brannan since he first became the editor of one of the best newspapers in the region. In fact, I had known him and worked with him for quite a while before we discovered that we shared something in common besides an incurable urge to write...

Diabetes.

That isn't surprising when you consider that good taste demands that one not boast about belonging to an exclusive group. After all, only about 10 percent of all Americans can qualify for membership. That is only slightly more than the number of Americans claiming to have had ancestors on the *Mayflower*.

I first learned of it when Dan wrote about a narrow escape from a bout of low blood sugar while driving down a winding mountain road. He was rescued by an alert young lady who wasn't above taking a few risks herself. He learned of my involvement with the malady when I delivered him a first-aid kit, consisting of some hard candy, after learning of his brush with disaster.

As a result of that experience – or maybe he planned to do it anyway – Dan, with great enthusiasm, was determined to write this book. He definitely aims to assure new people with diabetes, who have recently joined the club and entered a strange new world, that diabetes is *not* a death sentence and there is no reason a diabetic can't live a long and productive life.

You just have to learn to play the game under a new set of rules, and many of us think they are the rules *all* humans ought to be using anyway.

Read, enjoy and have a Happy, Healthy Life!

Carroll Gambrell
Walhalla, SC
July 1995

Prologue

Melanie Dawson was in her car near her Mountain Rest, S.C., home when she became involved in a potentially life-threatening situation for another person.

Dawson had been following a disoriented driver's truck in the Mountain Rest area for several miles and quickly became aware the driver was in trouble. She had several things go through her mind. Her first thought was that the person was on drugs or was drunk.

"I just kept praying that somehow I could get him to stop," she said.

Disregarding her own personal safety, she darted in front of the driver and forced him to stop. The person seemed dazed and confused upon her arrival.

She asked for his keys, which, thankfully, he handed over. At that point, Dawson still didn't know if the person was on drugs or was drunk.

The driver finally mumbled that he was a person with diabetes. Dawson knew the situation was serious. With the man's keys in her hand, she went down to a local convenience store and called for assistance. She was told to offer him orange juice to raise his blood sugar level.

Shortly after taking a few sips of orange juice, the person's sugar level began to return to normal and he snapped out of the daze. He had forgotten his lunch and worked out heavily, swimming nearly a half-mile and lifting weights. His sugar level had dropped so low that he was in insulin shock after he got in the car and attempted to return to work.

Dawson insisted the man go with her to the nearby convenience store and eat a sandwich. She continued to assist him and stayed with him until he was back to normal.

"I just like to help people, I guess," she told the man she had helped.

If Melanie had not stopped the driver, he would have continued into insulin shock and possibly lost consciousness. He could have easily crashed over the side of the mountain on the winding Mountain Rest road or hit another vehicle.

But thanks to the courage Melanie showed, the man was not

harmed and was able to make his return to reality unscathed.

I'm the man Melanie saved!

This incident woke me up to the seriousness of my disease. As one of the people profiled in this book, a man named Carroll Gambrell, says, "Once you become a person with diabetes, you enter a new world. The old world of eating chocolate cake anytime you pleased or going hours without eating if you pleased, or even getting intoxicated, are over. You have to carry food constantly and always be aware that you can drop low and can go into shock."

This book will show that you can live a relatively normal life with diabetes and be successful in whatever field you choose, whether it is being a newspaper editor, a novelist, a respected physician, a banker, a charity executive, a prison educator or even a professional athlete or musician. Different types of people are profiled in this book.

You will learn their personal stories - their struggles, successes, fears and hopes after being diagnosed with this disease. You will learn of the potentially deadly complications that can occur in any person with diabetes if a balance of diet, exercise and proper medication is not followed.

I hope also you will pay attention to the advice of the American Diabetes Association, the largest support group for persons with diabetes in the United States, and the Juvenile Diabetes Foundation. A portion of the proceeds from this book will go directly to the ADA and JDF. Every person with diabetes is in contact with the ADA or JDF.

There are so many ways to raise funds for diabetes research and education. Some are mentioned in this book. My favorite is South Carolina's Mountains-to-the-Sea run that begins in the South Carolina mountains and ends at the resort town of Myrtle Beach each Thanksgiving weekend.

The diabetic fraternity is 14 million strong in the U.S., but there are a total of 6-7 million cases that are undiagnosed. We must make ourselves aware of the disease and work to make others aware of diabetes and how it can be controlled. Diabetes was listed as the cause of death on 162,567 death certificates in 1990 in the U.S., which is more than died from AIDS in the same year. We must lobby to be treated as equals to those with AIDS and cancer in regard to federal funding. AIDS funding is considerably higher on the federal level even though more people die from diabetes-related complications.

We must find a cure for this disease.

With your help, we *will.*

CHAPTER 1

A Shattered Dream

I looked up and saw a nurse staring me in the face. She had a needle and a bottle of 70/30 Humulin-brand insulin.

It was showtime, time for my first self-administered shot.

I had always been terrified of needles. In fact, at that moment, I thought back to how I always fought to avoid the needle. I'd do anything not to take a shot. I don't know if a doctor or nurse had really botched a shot with me when I was a kid, but the fear was unbelievable. I saw my mom, who was frequently ill, injected constantly with needles and made myself a pledge - I'd rather die than take a lot of shots.

On this hot summer August day in Rocky Mount, N.C., I wondered if God had remembered that vow.

I had spent the last 24 hours psyching up for the moment. I

was all alone in that hospital.

My life had been one problem after another over the past year. The business I started was about to go belly-up. My wife, Terri, was already gone; she was preparing to have major back surgery in St. Louis, and the marriage's future was uncertain. I had financial problems galore. I had diabetes. And now I had to learn to inject insulin each day.

I had entered the hospital with a 700 blood sugar level. I was given insulin for several hours until the levels dropped. I broke out in a sweat when the level dropped to about 80 and had to eat something sweet to go back up. I remember shaking terribly while a pastor was in my room comforting me. I was sick to my stomach and felt confused. Finally, a nurse came in to assist me and gave me something to eat. The nurse didn't look at the sodas she selected and gave me a soda which was loaded with sugar.

Within minutes, my blood sugar level, which was already normal, had soared back up. And because of her error, I had to have another shot.

I was furious at that nurse. My first night in the hospital was horrible. I remember awakening about every three hours when the nurse would open the doors and look in at me. I even had to have an insulin shot at 4 o'clock the first morning.

I kept saying to myself, "Why me? Why me? Why do I have to have this horrible disease?"

Dr. John Mitchell, my doctor, had been highly concerned about me before I checked into the hospital. I shrugged it off, working up until the last minute. I didn't even bring my overnight bag when I went into the hospital. I remember that irritated Dr. Mitchell greatly.

I had always been so healthy before. How could Mr. Physical Fitness, Dan Brannan, possibly have a potentially life-threatening illness?

After waking up about 7 in the morning, I spent the next few hours jabbing a plastic object. It was supposed to simulate my body.

I always prided myself on a high degree of mind control. I told myself if I could keep my mind in the game to run two 26.2-mile marathons, I could give myself insulin shots.

The nurse was prepared for the big moment. She spread everything out on a table. The needle, insulin bottle and prep swabs were all there.

I said, pointing to a spot on my stomach, "Is this where I put the needle in?"

She looked back and said "Yes."

I said to her, "Do you realize how much I hate this?"

She looked back and said, "Yes, I sympathize, but then, maybe, I'll never know how it feels. You have to do this to get better."

With those words, I stuck the needle into my stomach and injected the insulin into my body.

Finally, after what seemed like an eternity, I was able to pull the needle out.

I had done it! I had given myself my first shot.

The hospital stay was awful. I'm afraid I don't make a good patient. I like to always be doing something, so sitting in a hospital bed watching TV and reading books was not a good way for me to pass the time.

The warning signs

The warning signs of diabetes for me were typical. I had all the symptoms – severe weight loss, fatigue, frequent urination, excessive thirst and ketones in my urine.

Thinking back, I think I was a person with diabetes for a pretty good while. I was really out of it one day when my boss came in, and I remember muttering something almost incoherently. I used to run at lunchtime. I remember coming back to work extremely thirsty and fatigued. I had a good friend on my staff who was a person with diabetes, and after observing me, felt that I possibly had the malady.

We made a bet that I could eat a chocolate cake and not be sick to my stomach. Somehow, we never finished the bet. I regret not going at that time and having myself checked out. I could have done some lasting damage to my system. I likely would not have gone into my own publishing company because the stress could have been too much. My illness was a big factor in the failure of my business.

I had a very successful career in the newspaper industry, serving as managing editor of two publications. I had been associated with a paper that had the country's highest percentage circulation increase in a six-month period in 1989. I had directed the Rocky Mount paper to historic circulation highs. I had won several state, regional and national honors while in Rocky Mount and was interviewed for two national publications, one in the

United States, the other in Canada.

I started my own publishing business in October 1993 after resigning from my position as managing editor of the Rocky Mount paper. It was a big risk, and the first few months were extremely tough. There was tremendous financial and emotional pressure.

Early in 1994, I could tell something was not right with me physically. I had to eat all the time to sustain energy. By February, I had no energy at all.

We published a 60-page special section that required nearly 72 hours of non-stop effort, and, I think, looking back on it, it may have pushed me over the edge. One day, I caught a glimpse of myself in the mirror and realized I looked terrible.

I was very thin; my weight had dwindled down to virtually nothing. I went from 180 pounds to 155 pounds. Each night, I woke up about every two hours to go to the bathroom.

Finally, I forced myself to go to a medical clinic and have myself checked out. I walked into the clinic knowing something was terribly wrong. I thought I either had diabetes, had AIDS or a form of cancer. Out of the choices, I hoped for diabetes.

I told the doctor's assistant of my suspicions. She opted to give me a urine glucose test, and I flunked. Next came a blood sugar test. My sugar level was more than 500. After Dr. Mitchell got the information, he came back with the verdict that I had diabetes.

I walked out of the clinic stunned. I tried not to cry, but I did. I remember sitting in my car in the doctor's parking lot and not knowing exactly what to do. I knew from that moment on I was going to be a person with diabetes the rest of my life. I already knew the consequences because my cousin had been a person with diabetes for years and my grandmother contracted diabetes late in life.

I was given stacks of material to read. I didn't really understand what I could eat. The doctors put me on Glucotrol pills to help control my diabetes.

At first, it seemed to help, but each time I went in for a blood sugar test, it seemed as though I couldn't get my levels down. We tried for a couple of months with the pills, using the highest dosage we could, but to no avail. We couldn't get the sugar level under control.

By this time, my weight had plunged to 143 pounds. I was starting to lose my hair and my business was in absolutely disastrous shape.

We had made a profit in March 1994, which was pretty incredible for the first six months of any business.

But in April, May and June, we lost several thousand dollars. I was unable to work efficiently, going in for a couple of hours and then having to go home and rest for another two hours before I could come back.

The diabetes had tremendously altered my physical appearance and practically destroyed it. My self-esteem was terrible. I couldn't get myself to go out in public, because every time I went out, I would see someone I knew.

They were absolutely alarmed at my weight loss and appearance. I even gave up several speaking engagements and work on community organizations because I felt so bad about my appearance. Instead, I would send one of my colleagues out to represent me.

My life continued to deteriorate in July 1994. My wife departed to have back surgery in the Midwest. My business was a disaster, continuing to amass severe losses. I had no more money left.

On Aug. 5, 1994, I entered Community Hospital in Rocky

Mount. Within 10 days after being hospitalized and receiving the necessary insulin, I had gained six pounds. Now the insulin was working properly in my system. One of my co-workers, seeing the weight I had gained back, joked with me that I must have been on steroids, I was looking so good.

I continued my improvement. My hair was growing back. By October, I had gained 20 pounds and I was offered an opportunity to serve as an editor for a pair of publications in Clemson and Seneca, S.C., that were planning to go daily.

I didn't want to leave my own business, for it had been my lifelong dream. I had worked and planned for my publishing company for two-and-a-half years prior to starting it.

Actually, it was something I had planned since my college days at Eastern Illinois University in Charleston, Ill. I could hardly stand giving it up, but I knew that if I didn't walk away, I would never really get healthy again. I was still struggling with fatigue.

I turned the business over to a partner, who did his best to keep it afloat, but we just didn't have enough capital to keep it going. Brannan Publishing, Inc., officially closed in December 1994.

My first days in the Seneca area were tough. I was so lonely and scared about my future. My wife was still not with me; in November 1994, she had her spinal fusion operation in St. Louis. I just made up my mind that things were going to be better, and somehow, I started to put myself back together, both financially and emotionally.

I was lucky to have made it out of Rocky Mount alive, as sick as I was. Thank God for insulin. Insulin was first developed in the early 1920s. Had I been born before the discovery, I probably wouldn't have lived for a year.

About a year after my hospitalization, my weight had gone from 143 to 187 pounds. I worked very hard over the year, swimming about two miles a week, running about 12 miles a week and lifting weights three days a week. I did nearly 1,000 situps each week.

I watched my diet, took my insulin regularly and tried to do everything the way I thought I should.

Over the last year-and-a-half, I've asked myself a million times "Why me? Why do I have diabetes? Do I deserve this?"

Each day, unless some new treatment is found, I'm going to have to inject myself with insulin just to live. I'll constantly have to test my blood sugar, go to the doctor and watch my diet. I realize the consequences could be devastating if I don't do everything I'm supposed to do.

As a person with diabetes, you have to learn how to take care of yourself, even if you have a spouse and other family members who love you. You have to watch out for yourself and avoid sweets, excessive alcohol, fatty foods and things that will hurt you.

Don't try to think it's something that's going to go away; it won't! You have entered a different world, one that will never be the same. Your life is forever different.

You just have to accept it and make the best of your life.

CHAPTER 2

The Family Link

Looking back, it is unbelievable how much experience I already had with diabetes.

The lifetime association began with my cousin Mike's diagnosis nearly a quarter of a century ago.

Mike had been a very sick child, suffering from asthma. He had been in and out of the hospital and was just beginning to improve with treatments, which included allergy shots and watching his diet.

When Mike was 7, my Aunt Martha believed he was showing some of the symptoms of diabetes. Aunt Martha had studied to be a nurse and had learned a lot about different illnesses. She took a specimen of Mike's urine to a local doctor's office in Carrollton, Ill.

Two days later, she said "We had our 7-year-old in Children's

Hospital in St. Louis."

"We were devastated. Mike had been so ill all of his life that we didn't know how we could handle this disease. We had been in the hospital with him so often with his asthma attacks. We all became involved in learning how to care for him and started treating him quickly. Children's Hospital had a very good program for (children with Type I diabetes)."

The Graners were involved in diabetes research at Children's Hospital for years. Mike went every summer for tests. Aunt Martha said she remembered one year, Mike had a very bad time and was in the hospital for a month of IV treatment. He also had severe problems with his left leg.

I remember when Mike went into the hospital for a month for the IV therapy. Everyone was so worried about him.

I was concerned he wouldn't make it out of the hospital. But he always did. He was a brave little fighter.

My mom had three sisters, Martha, Carole and Mary, along with a brother, Jim. Martha, Carole and Mary all lived close to us and between the four of them, had 11 children. I remember going on all kinds of picnics and family outings with the children. I also remember playing with Mike at my Aunt Carole's house. I always knew Mike had to be treated differently. He always carried a glucose tube with him everywhere he went. I remember Aunt Carole having to mark our plastic Kool-Aid cups with his name to ensure he got something that was sugar-free.

Aunt Carole said she and the rest of the family tried to learn what they could about diabetes once Mike developed the illness. Mike played in Aunt Carole's backyard and in the neighborhood on Fourth Street in Carrollton all the time.

"I kept orange juice in the refrigerator when he played out in the yard," said Aunt Carole. "If he ever had a reaction, he would come to the back door and ask for something to eat. I made sure I always had sugar-free soda for him in the refrigerator."

Three incidents that involved me with Mike stick out in my mind. I remember once, during high school track season, Mike's sugar started going low. We had become fairly close during the track season. I was a senior and co-captain of the track team. He was a freshman, but like I had done at the same age, made the varsity team. We trained together constantly and pushed each other, Mike competing in the half-mile and me the quarter.

I remember Mike falling on the ground during one of our

practice sessions. Thankfully, he knew what was going on and had glucose with him. He gave himself some and, in a few minutes, was OK.

I was scared to death. I asked him several times what to do when he was out of it, but he said all he needed was his glucose. At that point, I better understood what he had been dealing with all those years.

Three years later, I saw Mike drink alcohol for the first time. We were both attending a post-graduation party for his class at the time. I remember someone offering him a beer and he accepted a cup.

I said to him, "I didn't know you drank, Mike." I then asked, "Are you sure you can have that?"

Mike responded, "Yes, but if I ever do drink, I have to plan around it."

I didn't know exactly what he meant then. Today, I understand what he was saying: If someone with diabetes does drink alcohol, he or she must learn that alcohol contributes calories, yet may cause hypoglycemia. He also told me it was always necessary to drink in moderation. But it's always best not to drink at all.

A few years after graduation, Mike came to Shelbyville, Ill., one weekend to run the town's annual 10-kilometer (6.2-mile) road race. Mike, my cousin Gary, my sister Sharon and I all participated in the race.

Mike had always been legendary within our family for his eating prowess. He was known to consume a whole chicken. I remember after hearing this I was astounded. I usually would eat just two pieces.

After the Shelbyville race, I took everyone out for pizza. I couldn't believe how many pieces of pizza Mike consumed. I asked him, "How do you do it?" He said he had to eat a lot, as active as he was with his exercise regimen.

Again, I didn't understand why he always ate so much. Today, after developing diabetes, I do understand. Most of the time as a person with diabetes, and especially if you are not in tight control, you are hungry.

Right after my diagnosis, I would eat, eat and eat some more. Weight continued to fall off me because the food was not being stored in my body. I do not have that sense of hunger now, but if I have gone longer than four or five hours, or worked out vigorously, I am absolutely starved.

Martha and her husband, Bob, always encouraged Mike to accept his situation, test his sugar, take his insulin and exercise and diet.

"We are so proud of him," Martha said. "I have always felt because of his illness, he has gone into research. He has worked hard to get his Ph.D."

My grandmother, Paula Carmody, developed diabetes when she was 71 in 1979. She lived with the disease until her unexpected death Dec. 12, 1991. I remember seeing her death certificate and seeing diabetes listed as one of the causes of death. I think she would have lived much past 83 if it hadn't been for the illness. Aunt Carole agreed with me, saying the disease probably affected her blood vessels and helped cause the stroke which apparently killed her.

Aunt Carole said she recalls vividly when Grandma first developed the symptoms of diabetes.

"We were coming back from a shopping trip in Jerseyville and she said she was so dry," Aunt Carole explained. "There were other signs, too. She was extremely tired. I do especially remember her being thirsty as one of the signs."

Aunt Carole said my grandmother took medication to control the diabetes for several years, but eventually, she had to start taking insulin. Aunt Martha gave my grandmother her insulin shot every morning when she was available. Aunt Carole said my grandmother didn't enjoy giving herself shots, but could do it if Aunt Martha was out of town.

My grandmother apparently had a hard time sticking to the proper diet of a person with diabetes.

"She really loved sweets," said Aunt Carole. "It was very difficult for her not to eat sweets. She still splurged on sweets on occasion, even after she was diagnosed as a person with diabetes."

Aunt Carole worries about the diabetes continuing in the family. She said Mike's diagnosis, followed by my grandmother and my own discovery, have made her constantly more aware of herself possibly being a person with diabetes.

"I give a lot of thought to it," she said. "Every day is a battle for a person with diabetes to remain stable. If you don't remain stable, you can do damage to yourself."

Aunt Carole is right. Every day is a struggle for someone with diabetes. You can't overindulge in sweets and expect to stay healthy. You can't eat fatty foods, which push your cholesterol level high. You have to take your medication on time and exercise.

I worry about diabetes being passed along in my family in future generations. After my grandmother, the disease skipped the five children and hit two of the 13 grandchildren. I hear that often happens, although I don't know if there is any medical credence to it.

Only time will tell if diabetes does continue its path in my family. At least now, we will all automatically be on the lookout for the symptoms and hopefully not let the disease get out of hand before treatment occurs.

CHAPTER 3

Family Connections

═══════════

Mike Graner has a vivid memory of the day *diabetes mellitus* became an everyday word in our family.

He was just shy of his eighth birthday and lived on Fifth Street in quiet Carrollton, Ill, a 2,800-population farming community close to St. Louis and Springfield, Ill., the state capital.

"I didn't know anything about the disease at the time, so I took my cues from my parents," Mike said. "I remember my mom started crying after she told me. I began crying, too, without any real idea why. I suppose I figured it must be something serious. My dad, however, tried to calm us down, saying in effect that it wasn't the end of the world. He began naming off a number of people he knew who were diabetics and who were leading normal lives.

"I remember him mentioning a talented high school athlete

from Calhoun (Ill.). I believe he wanted me to know that diabetes wouldn't necessarily preclude my participation in sports. This was very important to me at the time, since I loved sports, basketball in particular.

"It was an emotionally spinning few minutes; there was this initial fear that I didn't understand - was I going to die? Why is Mom so upset? What's going to happen to me? My dad's 'litany of normalcy' quickly brought things back under control, and I began to slowly realize that things would be different for me, but that everything would be all right."

Mike was hospitalized for about a week at Children's Hospital in St. Louis, where he took part in a program run in conjunction with Washington University Medical School. Mike was then taught the mechanics of daily diabetic life: the now-archaic urine testing procedures, how and where to give shots and diet options.

He was also taught the background to diabetes, such as what was physiologically going on and what he could expect later. Their philosophy centered on teaching the patient how to monitor his or her condition and to make necessary adjustments through insulin, diet and exercise. Mike does not remember his first shot, probably because he had always been so sickly and had frequent shots, anyway.

Mike remembered, shortly after being diagnosed, talking to his best friend Mike Cronin about the disease, since he felt Mike could be trusted with the information.

"I guess I feared that I would be treated differently than the other kids, but I knew he would never do that to me," Mike said. "We were both only 7 at the time, so the implications of it were of little impact, and I'm sure we just went right on playing baseball or whatever. As it turns out, no one really treated me differently because I was diabetic, except perhaps to watch out for me a little more, or to try and have diet sodas around more often. Since that time, I've spoken to whoever wants to know about diabetes, what it means to me, and what it might mean to them. I don't go out of my way to bring it up in conversation, but I don't shy away from talking about it, either."

Mike remembers a couple of scares with his diabetes when he was a kid. One occurred when he was playing in a neighborhood church yard with Rob Lippert, another one of our cousins. Mike had only been diagnosed a few months before and was generally under good control, but that day, Mike began acting strangely and then fell to the ground, giggling incessantly. Rob started tickling Mike, not understanding he wasn't responding. Soon, Mike passed out entirely.

Rob ran for his mother (Aunt Mary) who called Mike's mother. She immediately came over to the yard and gave him some orange juice while someone else called an ambulance.

"I only remember playing baseball, then coming to in my dad's arms. I asked him why he was holding me, and then I noticed the ambulance and asked him who was hurt. It took me several minutes to become aware of what had happened. Being new to the diabetic signs of hypoglycemia, I must have not realized that my blood sugar had fallen that low, and I just kept on playing. I was very fortunate to have family that close by to respond."

The other incident occurred when Mike was attending St. John's Grade School in Carrollton. Mike had officiated a pre-lunch basketball game and went to lunch after that. He says the last clear memory he has of the event was leaving the building to go to the lunch room and thinking he was unbearably hungry.

"I have vague recollections of unsteadily walking around the edge of a concrete pit that was formerly a stairwell to a basement of an old school that had been torn down," said Mike. "Why I didn't fall in, I'll never know. I also hazily remember doing strange things in the lunch line, such as repeatedly moving my tray when the servers tried to put food on it. Once at the table, I apparently picked up another student, chair and all, and moved him over a space, saying that I wanted to sit in that spot. I also have this dream-like memory of people laughing at me as I ate a napkin. I must have been extremely hungry!

"The next relatively conscious memory I have was that of walking down the hall to the classroom, I figured out what had happened to me, and about that time the principal pulled me out of class to ask if I was OK, since students had told her I was acting very much out of character. There must have been some benefit to having a boring and predictable personality.

"To me, the most frightening aspect of that blood sugar crash was that it happened so quickly that I didn't notice the warning signs, and by then, I certainly knew what they were."

Mike's parents, Bob and Martha, never let him feel he'd brought any type of grief to their lives and always strived to treat him like any other normal person.

"Of course, there were additional responsibilities to deal with because of the diabetes, such as preparing or weighing food portions, learning exchanges or helping with the shot rotation," Mike said. "My folks never showed any signs that the extra work bothered them; it was just another aspect of raising me.

"I think their ability to make these lifestyle changes run so smoothly led to my attitude toward my diabetes, that it is a part of my life that I cannot, I must not, ignore, but it does not run my life for me."

Mike says he didn't feel different from other teen-agers because of his diabetes. Most of his friends never made any issue of the things he had to do. For Mike, it was just a matter of making adjustments for odd eating times or quantities and unusual sleep patterns.

"High school sports were sometimes a problem, since our practices were quite demanding and often, I was in need of carbohydrates and water, but our coaches at least gave me free rein to take care of myself. Socially and psychologically, I did not suffer because of the disease."

People have often asked Mike if he doesn't hate having to take shots every day. His response is, "Of course, I don't enjoy it, but the fact that it keeps me alive somehow makes it tolerable."

Mike has been an inspiration. In grade school, he was a star basketball and track athlete. In high school, he played football all four years and excelled in track. He attended the University of Illinois and today has his doctorate. He is a scientist, working at the University of Arizona's Department of Molecular and Cellular Biology in Tucson, Ariz.

Mike controls his diabetes by taking four shots a day, which he calls "the poor man's insulin pump." He takes a mixture of regular and NPH insulin in the morning, regular insulin at lunch and dinner, and NPH again in the evening. His dosages are pretty low on a per-kilogram body-weight basis. He attributes this to exercise. Mike and I are firm believers that exercise is vital to the regimen of a person with diabetes.

Mike used to make the long-distance runs on the dusty country roads buried between our hometown cornfields. I remember seeing Mike out on long runs, either going back or on his way out. It was actually kind of funny. Mike, my sister Sharon and my cousins Gary Kesinger and Rob Lippert and I could all be found trotting around on those roads training while we were in high school and even in the post-high school years.

In graduate school, Mike's athletic interests turned to weight training. He dabbled in rugby for a while, then returned to a focus on weight training in recent years.

Mike's diet is largely fruit-based; he eats a lot of bananas, with a great deal of skim milk. He says he also enjoys raw vegetables and eats mainly grilled chicken when he eats any type of meat.

Mike feels fortunate to have no major physical complications due to his diabetes, even though he has had the illness for 25 years.

"I would like to think that by maintaining good control of my diet and doing whatever else I can to stay healthy will result in a normal lifespan and one that is free of complications," Mike said. "However, I don't know that I can make those assumptions. The thought of retinopathy or kidney disease, and the host of other problems that are associated with diabetes, frightens me, and it's not entirely clear that 'clean living' will prevent the complications in all cases.

"Nonetheless, if it comes down to some form of a diabetic Pascal's wager, I will work hard to keep healthy and my life under control. At the very least, I feel better when my control is good. In another sense, I cannot devote excessive time and energy worrying about potentially impending complications, provided I'm doing my best to avoid them now. The chips will fall where they may, and wherever they do fall, I'll accept it and work from there."

Mike feels very lucky in many respects. "It's not fun having diabetes, but I guess there are worse fates in life," he told me. "While I've always realized I was somewhat different, I've never felt alone, weird or excruciatingly unusual. I'm healthy, and the precepts of diet and exercise for diabetic living have undoubtedly contributed to that, and would benefit anyone's life.

"For me, diabetes has never been the major issue in my existence; it's just been a part of me that required daily attention. Maybe the way I saw my parents deal with it, or it may be my own personality quirks made my attitude what it is. Diabetes is not the end of the world. It is a sometimes strange and frightening trip into realms of self-awareness, but I think having diabetes has led me to learn and understand things about myself that I might never have explored had I not had the disease. I think diabetes is part of the reason why I'm a scientist today. I also think it has been a basal force driving me to stay in shape. I've been in good control most of my life, and I've had expert help doing that.

I just hope it continues."

Mike and I have been away from each other for several years. Somehow, now, I feel closer to him than ever before. Maybe it's because we share this disease.

I also feel I better understand what he and his family went through when he was growing up. I better understand the fear they went through when he was first diagnosed and all the work that went into making Mike the person he is today.

CHAPTER 4

A Diabetes Primer

Diabetes is one of those diseases that, by its very definition, can positively chill the living daylights out of anyone.

Diabetes (officially *diabetes mellitus*) is a chronic metabolic disorder that adversely affects the body's ability to manufacture and/or utilize insulin, a hormone necessary for the conversion of food into energy.

Normally, with the help of insulin (a hormone made in the pancreas), the cells use sugar for energy or store it for later use.

But in people with diabetes, insulin is either lacking (absent or reduced) or is not effective. In either case, the cells are unable to make use of the sugar, which collects in the blood and eventually in the urine. The treatment for diabetes aims to keep blood-sugar levels in the near-normal range, with hopes of preventing complications.

There are two major types of diabetes – Type I, or insulin-dependent, diabetes, and Type II, or non-insulin dependent, diabetes.

People with Type I diabetes require insulin injections each day to stay alive. They are commonly diagnosed from infancy to their late 30s. People with Type II diabetes often come down with it in their middle or later years; the insulin is often present, but not used properly. Treatment procedures involve dietary and weight control and oral medications; injections may be required in some cases. An estimated 14 million Americans, and 120-125 million worldwide, have this disease.

A total of 90 percent of all diagnosed diabetes cases are Type II; surprisingly, some of people with Type II diabetes *do* require injections. The remaining 10 percent of cases are Type I diabetes.

Diabetes is listed as one of the main causes of death worldwide because of the complications. The Centers for Disease Control in Atlanta reported 162,567 people had diabetes or its complications listed on their death certificates in 1990. That figure had grown enormously from 135,931 in 1980.

There are numerous complications of this disease. Here are

some to think about:

- Cardiovascular disease is 2-4 times more common in people with diabetes than in those who do not have the disease.

- The incidence of strokes is 2-6 times higher for people with diabetes.

- Hypertension, or high blood pressure, affects 60-80 percent of all people with diabetes.

- The death rate from kidney disease is 500 times higher in young adults with diabetes than in those who do not have it.

- Blindness caused by diabetes changes the lives of as many as 24,000 people each year; it is also the leading cause of new cases of adult blindness each year in the United States, costing $75 million a year in federal and state aid.

The comprehensive U.S. national cost of diabetes - including hospital, nursing home and physician care, laboratory tests, pharmaceutical products, and patient workdays lost because of disability and premature death - totals more than $100 billion each year.

Type I warning signs are frequent urination, including frequent bedwetting in children who have been toilet-trained; sudden weight loss; excessive thirst; extreme hunger; weakness and fatigue; and irritability.

Type II warning signs include any of the just mentioned warning signs, plus blurred vision or any change in sight; slow healing of cuts, especially on the feet; frequent infections; tingling or numbness in legs, feet or fingers; and frequent skin infections or itchy skin.

However, many people with Type II diabetes have no symptoms at all. In fact, for every person with known Type II diabetes, there is another person who has it, but does not know it.

An emphasis is now being made by the American Diabetes Association to get individuals to look at their family history. Della Kelley, a technical information specialist for the Centers for Disease Control in Atlanta, says the number of people with diabetes is increasing across the country. It is still, however, mostly a disease of older people.

"Our population is aging," Kelley said. "Diabetes in young people is much different than it is in older people. For younger people, the type of diabetes they get is Type I, or insulin-dependent, and most of them cannot live without insulin. It is usually a sudden onset for them.

"Ninety to 95 percent of those people, diagnosed and undiagnosed and depending on their bodies, do not produce enough insulin, but it's not as much a problem as it might be for another person. Those people can be treated by monitoring their diet and exercising regularly. Many of them, however, will ultimately use insulin."

I was one of those persons. My diabetes may have existed for a long time before I even felt sick with it. The doctors I interviewed for this book have told me you can have diabetes for as long as eight years before the first visible symptoms ever become known.

Believe it or not, however, I share the disease with many famous people. The list of celebrities with diabetes is a long and distinguished one. They include Hall of Fame baseball pitcher Jim "Catfish" Hunter; Hall of Fame hockey player Bob Clarke; NFL quarterback Wade Wilson; actress Mary Tyler Moore; former Soviet Union premier Mikhail Gorbachev; country music singer Mark Collie; rock music singer Bret Michaels; and many, many others.

You'll be reading stories of people with diabetes throughout this book. Despite how horrible this disease can be, all of them have vowed to fight on and be examples of how to triumph over diabetes, not the other way around.

Their stories are inspiring to anyone; I know they inspired me.

CHAPTER 5

You Are What You Eat

Just after my diagnosis of being a person with diabetes, I made a trip to the grocery store.

I will never forget it as long as I live. I remember walking into the Winn-Dixie store near my home in Rocky Mount, N.C. The Winn-Dixie was my favorite store because it was not only close, but had a great selection of items.

I remember getting a cart and heading to aisle No. 1. Suddenly, a tremendous sense of fear came over me. I thought to myself, "What exactly can I buy?" I thought of my meal plan and tried to think about the items I needed to purchase.

I went through a few items and, remembering what the dietitian had preached, I checked for grams of sugar and grams of fat. It seemed every item I picked up had too much sugar.

Pulling into aisle No. 2, I had only one thing in the cart. As

I pushed the cart down the second aisle, my frustration continued to build. By the time I reached the third aisle, I had only a few things in the cart. Tears started rolling down my face. I tried to hide my head where no one could see me. I kept saying to myself, "Why me, God? What did I do to deserve this? What in the world can I eat? How am I going to handle all this by myself?"

I hurried and got through the store and completed my trip. I remember my total bill was a whopping $15.

I went back home and read everything I could get my hands on about what a person with diabetes could eat. Next, I made a list, and the following day, went back to the store. During my first several doctor's visits, I asked a lot of questions about my diet.

It has taken me a long time to become comfortable with my diet. Even recently, I made a discovery after glucose testing that will likely help in years to come.

I ate about four pieces of one of the new stuffed-crust pizzas out on the market, then tested my sugar. The reading was 339 points, which floored me. The next day, I called a diabetes educator at the local hospital and asked her about it.

She told me she believed it was the fats in the sausage, pepperoni and possibly the sauces that had pushed my sugar up. She told me it would be best to order a thin-crust cheese pizza and only eat a couple of pieces.

I couldn't believe this - I had to give up pizza loaded with sausage, pepperoni and beef. I thought to myself, "Is there anything that is fun that I can eat?"

One of my good friends made me a homemade pizza recently with Ragu Light sauce, which has no sugar added and contains only 5 grams of natural sugars. I am thankful pizza will not have to be totally excluded from my diet; I'll just have to remember eating this way will help to preserve my health.

Making changes in my diet was one of the toughest things about becoming a person with diabetes. I loved peanut butter and honey sandwiches. I gave up those more than a year ago. I liked cereals with more sugar in them. I have traded one brand of cereal for another brand which has only 1 gram of sugar; eating them with a banana peeled on top has helped them become more palatable for me.

I have pretty much stopped eating frozen yogurt, although Eskimo Pie is my favorite, which has only about 5 grams of sugar; you should always check the labels, however, for sugar content.

I keep my diet pretty much the same every day unless I eat out or travel. I eat six times a day, following a 3,000-calorie diet because of my athletic lifestyle.

Breakfast for me is usually Cheerios and a banana. I eat crackers and low-fat cheese for a mid-morning snack, then eat fresh turkey, low-fat cheese and lettuce and tomato on a sandwich with an apple for lunch. I eat half a sandwich of turkey or chicken at about 3 p.m., then some chicken or fish, baked potatoes or salad for supper. I normally eat half a turkey sandwich for my nighttime snack. Sometimes, I eat popcorn.

I always look at every item I purchase in the grocery store for sugar and fat content. I ask a lot of questions when I eat out. I remember one time in the spring I ate with my dad and sister's family at an Italian restaurant. I wanted what they were having so badly, and after asking questions, I was able to have it. If I hadn't asked the questions, they wouldn't have made my dinner without adding sauce with sugar and my blood sugar would have shot up.

Dr. John Colwell is an M.D., Ph.D, and professor of medicine as well as being the director of the Diabetes Center at the Medical University of South Carolina in Charleston. He was mentioned as one of the top experts in the world on diabetes by *Town and Country* magazine and is recognized among his peers nationally and internationally as an expert on diabetes and its vascular complications.

Colwell is a stickler about a saturated-fat restricted diet for patients with diabetes.

"You have to get the right carbohydrate-protein-fat balance to get the optimum mix in a diet plan," he said. "The diet also should be 30 percent and less in fat and modest in protein. Fruit, vegetables and grains are best to have in the diet. Dietary fiber is also important."

Colwell explained that for those with Type II diabetes, diet and exercise are equally important. People with Type II diabetes control their illness primarily by what they eat and exercising.

Dr. Frank Axson is an internist in my current hometown of Seneca, S.C., who treats many people with diabetes in this part of the country. About 20 percent of the patients who visit his internal medicine practice are those with diabetes. He says diet is most important to the success in treating his patients.

"I remember a physician at Emory, S.C., once said that 90 percent of the people would be off insulin if they were on a proper diet," Axson said. "Perhaps his expectations are awfully high, but I believe a good many people with diabetes could get off insulin if they did follow the right diet. A person with diabetes has to watch fats and get calories down. Total calories are much more important than anything else in a the diet of a person with diabetes. Meats, desserts, dairy products such as eggs and a lot of the salad dressings, should be restricted for someone with diabetes."

Dr. Rob Lindemann and Cindy Floyd, a certified diabetes educator, are in agreement that counting carbohydrates is the best thing a person with diabetes can do about his or her diet.

"The American Diabetes Association issued new standards of care in December 1994, and part of those standards had to do with sugars and carbohydrate counting," said Floyd. "A diabetic's 15 grams of carbohydrate counting can come from anywhere."

The common myth is that persons with diabetes can't have anything with sugar. That has been proven incorrect. However, carbohydrates do need to be counted.

"Carbohydrate counting is the best way to do the diet overall," said Lindemann. "Persons with diabetes need a balanced diet with no more than 30 percent of calories from fats. A standard to follow is a 50 percent carbohydrate, 30 percent protein and 20 percent fat diet. No medicine precludes a proper diet, exercise and weight control for a person with diabetes. Today, we recognize that the diet of a person with diabetes can be a lot more flexible."

Floyd is seeing that the insulin intake of those with Type I diabetes is dependent on their carbohydrate counting.

"Patients should follow the ADA's exchange list diet and the diet prescribed to them by their doctor," said Floyd. "Adults typically don't need a high-protein diet, unless they are athletes. Unfortunately, most adults are basically sedentary."

If you have Type I diabetes, more frequent doses of insulin will allow more diet flexibility. My plan is to move toward more shots a day for that luxury.

For Type IIs, following the proper diet and exercise plan may be just what is necessary to stay away from daily insulin shots.

All persons with diabetes should stay in tune with the ADA's recommendations on dietary guidelines and frequently consult with their doctor, diabetes educators and dietitians.

They say you are what you eat. For a person with diabetes, your survival and the key to a long, successful life is your diet.

CHAPTER 6

New Frontiers of Treatment

The key to the treatment process for persons with diabetes is a simple one: Close monitoring of your blood sugar level and tight control of your diet and levels once treatment begins.

I have to admit I made many mistakes since I was diagnosed with diabetes. The first mistake I made was staying on oral medications too long. My doctor in Rocky Mount, N.C., probably had wanted me to go on insulin several days before I actually did, but I fought insulin injections tooth and nail.

You really couldn't blame me; like most people, the thought of having to stick needles inside myself every day in order to live was, at best, a chilling one. Problem was, the oral medication didn't work for me.

Once I started taking shots, I made nearly an immediate turnaround. I gained most of my weight back in a few months and felt, as Dr. Mitchell said I would, "better and stronger than I have in years."

I guess my first piece of advice for a person with diabetes is not to fight insulin injections if that treatment is what you need. Believe it or not, somehow, you do get adjusted to jabbing yourself with needles every day.

Hey, if Dan Brannan, who was probably more scared of needles than anyone in the world, can give himself injections, you can, too. Hopefully, you will join the majority who have Type II diabetes not requiring insulin injections, but instead, maintain themselves through oral medication, diet and exercise, instead of insulin.

The key thing in the beginning is to establish yourself with a doctor who is knowledgeable about diabetes. In cases such as mine, it is recommended that one finds an internist who specializes in the disease.

A complete physical should be performed and the doctor should make sure no damage has been done to the eyes, kidneys, nerves, cardiovascular system and vascular area because of the previously untreated diabetes.

In the beginning, I went to the doctor about once a week.

After moving to Seneca, S.C., I waited several weeks before I found a doctor. I believe that was a big mistake, as well.

Another error: I was only testing my sugar once every few days. I should have realized that there is no way you can monitor your diabetes by not checking your blood sugar two to three times daily.

For several months, I was taking 50 units of Humulin-type insulin each morning. Cindy Floyd, a certified diabetes educator mentioned later in the book, showed me this type of medication process would not work for someone as active as I am.

Cindy explained that the Humulin I was taking had a 12-hour lifespan. That is, if I was taking it at 6 a.m. each day, it would be completely out of my system by 6 that evening.

After talking to my doctor, Dr. Billy Campbell in Westminster, S.C., he recommended that I go to a second shot. Floyd said an even better way to treat the diabetes is to do it much like my cousin Mike is doing, taking injections 3-4 times a day and mixing types of insulin. You do have to be very careful when mixing insulin, though, to take it on time and at the same time each day; in other words, to establish a schedule and stick to it, no matter what.

Through Cindy, I have very much relearned the importance of testing. I wasn't totally aware of some of the figures I should strive for in terms of my blood-sugar level. A patient's goal should be 150 milligrams per deciliter of blood at all times. Normal fasting levels are 70-120 mg/dl. Anytime the sugar level of a person with diabetes creeps past 200 mg/dl, it should set off alarms in a person's head. If it goes above 250, then ketone testing should be performed immediately.

A key advancement has been the hemoglobin-A1c test, which tests a patient's sugar level over a six-week period. A person with diabetes has seen treatment devices progress from 24-hour urine collections to electronic devices, which allows you to test blood outside the machine. Needles are much finer and sharper today, and we even have syringes that are disposable and thinner than they used to be. The insulin pump has also come into use in this country (it has been available internationally for some time now) and also promises to be a major factor in the treatment of diabetes.

The key thing to remember is that if your blood-sugar level goes too low, which is below 60 mg/dl, to drink 4 ounces of orange juice or regular cola or chew a couple of peppermint candies or other hard candy. Symptoms of a low level include tremors, a fast heartbeat, tingling, nausea, headache, dizziness and staggering. After the symptoms go away, eat a light meal, such as a glass of milk, a meat sandwich or a peanut butter sandwich.

Dr. Rob Lindemann sees Glucometers as a major part of the treatment process of a person with Type I or Type II diabetes. "The day-to-day measures are very important," Lindemann said. "It's important to continue on that day-to-day basis."

People who are on only one dose of insulin, unless they live in a shell, are not in very good control, Lindemann believes. "No person's pancreas produces the same amount of insulin day-to-day," he said. "A lot of physicians do not understand that concept. When you take 2-3 shots a day and test 2-3 times a day, you usually have more flexibility over what you can eat."

Dr. John Colwell said technology has moved along very well in glucose testing. He says the hemoglobin-A1c testing window has made it a lot easier to detect how patients are doing. "Everyone is trying to work out different systems of assessing blood sugar control," Colwell said. "Sticking your finger 5-6 times a day does get old after awhile, but it is necessary for intensive diabetes management."

Mike Muir, my pharmacist at The Medicine Shoppe in Seneca, S.C., has watched the meters go all the way from $800 to less than $50 today - with rebate. "The test strips are what cost you, and they run for about $30 for a bottle of 50 these days," Muir said.

It's very important to develop a strong relationship with your local pharmacist. I've even called Mike when I needed insulin as late as 12:50 p.m., 10 minutes before closing time on Saturday; and he waited for me. Mike has searched the country over for swabs for me because I didn't like the very moist types of swabs (I seemed to bruise easier when I used them), and he found some medium-range swabs for me to use.

Mike is the type of pharmacist who will also take time for those who have diabetes and explain the various medications and treatment devices. He understands how the various testing devices work and also offers highly competitive prices. To me, Mike Muir is the ideal pharmacist and a good friend. Mike is not in his business just to make a buck. He sincerely cares about his patients and is a true family pharmacist.

I currently use the Advantage type of digital tester. I've also had a One-Touch tester, which provided previous readings for me. I prefer the Advantage system, though, because it tests the blood on the outside and it is easier to get the blood on the strip.

My fingers do get sore sometimes from testing; after all, I have to draw blood 3-4 times a day. I've gotten into the habit of testing at regular intervals during the day.

Another important aspect of a pharmacist is that he'll look out for you when it comes time to purchase cold medicines or other types of over-the-counter drugs and point out what has sugar and what doesn't, such as cough medicines, laxatives and other types of medications and drugs.

For those with Type II diabetes, there is a new medication on the market called Glucophage. Muir says this medication may keep some patients from having to go to injections because it is a stronger form of oral medication with a unique mode of action.

In any case, tight control is the key, and the only way that will happen is through the right kind of medication, constant testing, watching your diet and exercising.

If you haven't seen a doctor in several weeks and have just been diagnosed, don't hesitate – go choose one immediately and schedule an appointment as quickly as possible. Diabetes will always be there; it's not like having a cold or chicken pox, knowing it will go away sooner or later.

The quicker you get yourself to a doctor, the easier your treatment may be and the more you will know about how to take care of yourself.

CHAPTER 7

Work That Body

On my way out of the hospital on Aug. 6, 1994, I was forced by hospital personnel to sit and be pushed out in a wheelchair by a nurse.

"It's hospital policy," said the nurse. "All patients have to be taken out by wheelchair when they check out."

I thought it was absurd, but I obliged. I'll get my revenge in just a few minutes, I silently told myself.

I went to my pickup truck, unlocked the back and put all my stuff in. My suitcase was loaded with materials and supplies. But what a sight my red gym bag was, loaded with swimming goggles, cap and swim trunks.

Now it was time for my revenge. I drove out of the hospital parking lot and headed for the Rocky Mount, N.C., Downtown YMCA. It was time to start exercising again.

I swam 500 yards without stopping and felt pretty good. The insulin was already starting to affect me. Next, I ran about two miles, then lifted weights for about 15 minutes. When I finished all this, I rode a bike for a mile and a half. This was all just after leaving the hospital.

I have always been a fitness buff. The exercise addiction began when I was 18 years old as a second-semester college freshman. I concluded my first semester with about 20 pounds of extra girth on my body. I decided that wouldn't work and started running, then added weightlifting to the regimen.

I have always exercised since then, running a lot of 10-kilometer (6.2-mile) races. I finished the 26.2-mile Monticello, Ill., Freedom Marathon in October 1983 in 3 hours, 58 minutes, then ran another marathon in Richmond, Va., in October 1991, in 4 hours, 45 minutes.

The swimming regimen came into play after a weekend trip to Atlantic Beach, N.C., with my sister, Sharon. Sharon had started swimming seriously a few years before that. I admired her for being able to compete in triathlons. It's kind of funny; I had gotten her into running about 10 years before. She returned that favor by taking me to the beach and swimming all day long. During the day, she explained how good it felt to swim all the time. The following Monday, we went to the YMCA and tried the pool out. I was able to go back and forth just a few times, but I loved it. I was hooked.

Today, I swim two miles a week, going 700 meters two days a week; 650 two days; and 500 on another. I also run two miles six days a week; lift weights lightly for 20 minutes three times a week; and do about 1,000 situps each week.

Who knows, maybe that addiction delayed the progress of my diabetes. One of the doctors I interviewed for the book told me medical experts do believe it is possible for someone to have diabetes for as long as eight years before exhibiting strong symptoms.

I have always wanted to compete in the Gatorade Ironman Triathlon in Kona, Hawaii. There have been several athletes with diabetes who have completed the Ironman, which consists of a 2.4-mile swim, a 112-mile bike ride and a 26.2-mile run.

Dr. Bob Laird has been medical director of the Ironman for the past 13 years. I decided to give him a ring because I wanted to show other people with diabetes there are no limits to what they can accomplish athletically and also reinforce the importance of aerobic exercise through things like running, swimming and walking.

What amazes Laird is that people with diabetes need little, if any, insulin during the day to complete the rigorous Ironman course.

"The exercise negates their need for insulin," he said. "I have never seen a person with diabetes have a problem in the Ironman. By the time they get here, they have done so much training and are so much in tune with their bodies they know what to do at all times. Athletes who are diabetics are so aware of their bodies. They don't allow themselves to get into trouble. To me, it's not surprising people with diabetes do well once they get here. Most who come here are relatively young and in good shape and maintain tight control on their blood sugar."

Bill Carlson has fared very well in Ironman competition and is a person with diabetes. He is the only person with diabetes with an insulin pump to finish the race.

Laird says exercise is extremely important, not only for those with diabetes, but anyone.

"It has a big psychological impact as well as helping the regulation of insulin," Laird said.

I told Laird of my daily runs and swims and he gave me a personal invitation to participate in the Ironman someday. I have set a goal that I will by age 40, but we will have to see.

For those who have spent the past several years curled up as couch potatoes, get off the couch. Of course, clear with your physician what kind of exercise routine is good for a beginner.

People with diabetes have to exercise to stay completely healthy. Exercise will burn off sugar and help in the use of insulin and medication. An excellent way for someone sedentary to begin an exercise program is by walking. You could start with a 10-minute walk, then build up to 30 minutes; check with a doctor before starting.

Swimming, my favorite, is also excellent. At first, a few laps would suffice, then over time, more laps could be added. I love to do situps and think everyone should to keep a trim waist. Starting with 10-20 situps would be a great beginning.

Dr. Frank Axson agreed with Laird that everyone, not just those with diabetes, should exercise a minimum of 30 minutes three times a week.

"Diet, medication and exercise have to coincide each day for a diabetic to be perfectly healthy," said Axson.

Dr. Colwell said exercise creates insulin sensitivity and increases the chances of the drug working effectively in the body.

"A lot of Type IIs can control their diabetes with the right diet and exercise," Colwell said. "Exercise lowers the cardiovascular risks in people with diabetes. It is good to exercise consistently three or four times a week."

Dr. Lindemann remembered a recent study which supported the importance of exercise for people with diabetes.

"One study showed people who were at higher risks resisted exercise, while those who exercised had a much lower incidence of risk," said Lindemann. "Aerobic exercise is really important. It is good to work out 30-40 minutes three to four times a week, if not on a daily basis, with a low impact aerobic routine."

The key to maintaining an exercise program is establishing a routine. It has to become a daily part of your life. Set a goal, then achieve it. If you say today I'm going to run for 30 minutes, don't settle for less.

I've found the best times for a workout are the very first thing in the morning and at lunchtime. By evening, I am usually just completely worn out. It is better to run or walk in the morning and work out in a gym or swim at lunch because the temperatures are normally up by noon.

One thing to remember is to carry a piece of candy or enough glucose to treat hypoglycemia and identification with you when running or walking.

One day, I was running with a good friend. About halfway through the run, I stumbled and fell. It was extremely hot out; we had waited until about 10 o'clock on a blazing hot July morning in South Carolina to run. I had already taken insulin and was already tired from the night before. After stumbling, I started to run again and fell down again, this time to my knees.

My friend walked me into the shade and sat with me, worried to death. I had a blank expression on my face and was headed into insulin shock. The friend then waved a truck down; the driver took us to my house, which was only about a quarter of mile down the road. Without the friend's help, I doubt if I could have made it home.

My friend had to trick me into drinking orange juice. I didn't know anything was wrong. Shortly after a few sips of orange juice and a sandwich, I was OK.

I learned another valuable lesson from that incident. I always keep a piece of candy in my shoe when I run to have in case something happens.

I encourage any person with diabetes who is not exercising to take the plunge, but be careful. You will feel better both mentally and physically. The only way to exercise regularly is to establish a routine.

Establishing a daily exercise routine may prevent damage to your organs and keep you healthy for the rest of your life.

I guarantee you will feel better if you bite the exercise bullet!

CHAPTER 8

Suffer The Children

════════════

Meloney Stokes is a mother and a housewife in Seneca, S.C.

Back in May 1993, Stokes had a very traumatic experience, one that would change her life, her husband Jim's and her entire family's, especially her youngest son, Justin.

Before that month, Justin had been the typical 3-year-old, but during a weekend, Justin fell ill – very ill. He spent the weekend lying around, something that was most unusual for such an active child. Justin would get up, then go right back to bed. This pattern continued for the entire weekend.

Thinking Justin had some sort of virus, Meloney decided to take Justin to the doctor that Monday. Surprisingly, during the weekend, Justin had turned down some Kool-Aid and chocolate cake, but Meloney really didn't think anything unusual about that.

That Monday afternoon, they went to the doctor's office.

Upon examination, the doctor said Justin's throat was very red and suspected what Meloney had thought, that Justin had a virus. Then Meloney told the doctor Justin had lost a lot of weight and consumed sugared drinks all the time.

She told the doctor to take a look at Justin's back, which seemed to be bony.

The doctor asked Meloney if Justin went to the bathroom often. Meloney responded, "Yes, he goes all the time."

Justin was given a urine test by the doctor. When the test results were analyzed, the doctor stated, "I think Justin has diabetes."

Meloney and Jim nearly fell to the floor in shock. Additional tests were performed, and they confirmed what the doctor had thought: Justin was, indeed, a person with diabetes.

The lives of the entire Stokes family were about to change.

Justin entered the hospital with a blood-sugar level of 688, meaning Justin had to begin taking insulin injections.

That didn't exactly sit too well with Justin, as one might expect with any 3-year-old. After all, who in their right minds would want to have to stick themselves with a needle every day in order to live?

Justin's parents had to plead with him many times to take his shot. Eventually, Justin submitted, but it wasn't easy. Today, of course, things have changed; Justin takes shots at 7 a.m., 6 p.m. and 11 p.m. daily and tests his blood sugar 4-5 times each day.

He still doesn't like the idea of having to stick himself with needles to live. "It's dumb and it just sucks," he has said to his mother.

His mother agrees. "It's an unfair disease," she said. "You have to take in account everything from diet to how hot it is. It's very difficult."

In the fall of 1994, Meloney and Jim had a scare with Justin. He had eaten nine cookies from a bag that had been labeled as having no grams of sugar.

Wrong! The cookies turned out to have seven grams of sugar, and having eaten nine cookies, this was seven grams and nine cookies too much for him.

Shortly after eating them, Justin became very ill. His sugar level rose dramatically, then plunged just as drastically, bottoming out at a level of 34 points. Throughout the night, Justin got up several times to throw up. Finally, at 7 the next morning, his parents took him to the hospital, where he spent several hours before being discharged.

After the incident, Meloney made contact with the cookie company, and after discussing what had happened, the company realized there had been an error in printing the nutritional information. Corrections immediately went out, but the cookie company declined to pull its products off the shelf.

Meloney immediately contacted a local attorney, who said she would have to fight the battle to get the cookies recalled herself. In response, Meloney called the Food and Drug Administration in Washington and the news department of Greenville, S.C., television station WYFF-TV. Both of them showed up at the Stokes' house on the same day. The station aired her story later that day, a Friday. By the following Monday, the cookies had been taken off the shelf.

Soon, however, Meloney realized that for kids like Justin, there was no support group or any other group that could help him realize he wasn't the only kid in the world who had come down with diabetes. She decided to form a support group for children with diabetes and their parents in Oconee County, S.C., where the Stokes family lives.

This group has attracted many children with diabetes and their parents since it was formed in 1995. "We don't want it to be a war-story type of thing," Meloney said, "but we just want to make sure our kids aren't treated differently from other kids.

"It will be good for the kids to see other children who have diabetes, too."

Despite the seriousness of the disease, Meloney realizes that there is no point in trying to hide the disease from other people. "We don't hide it when it's time for him to take his shots," she said. "Everyone is very comfortable with the fact he has to inject himself, and everyone at his school knows he is a person with diabetes, but he's not treated any differently from other kids."

The Stokes want Justin to do anything he wants to in his life. Justin says he doesn't exactly know what he wants to do, but he thinks he would like to be an ice skater.

Whatever Justin wants to be, he will more than likely accomplish it, given his parents' support and his strong iron will.

CHAPTER 9

...And a Teen Will Lead Them

One look at Katie Plemmons will make the average male's heart beat a little faster.

Katie has it all. Great looks. Sparkling personality. A brain that matches her beauty.

Oh, and one other thing: Katie has diabetes.

Katie lives in Roanoke, Va., and was first diagnosed as a person with diabetes when she was 6 years old. "I had a virus," she said, "and before I knew it, all the symptoms came crashing down on me. I was thirsty all the time, and every time I drank a Coke, I became thirstier."

Her family had a ketone test performed on her, and as things turned out, Katie was spilling an incredible amount of the substance in her urine.

Further tests were performed. They confirmed her family's

worst fears: Katie had diabetes.

When the word came through, her mother, Judy (who is a nurse) immediately took Katie to the hospital as soon as she got home from school. "My first insulin shot was in my leg," she recalled. "I remember staring at the needle the whole time. It was very scary."

Growing up with diabetes has not been the easiest thing to do. Like many others with diabetes, Katie has had her ups and downs. At age 12, things suddenly caved in on her. She had trouble maintaining her blood-sugar level and had to obtain an insulin pump to help her maintain her levels properly.

One time, while at a cheerleading contest in Cocoa Beach, Fla., a combination of bad insulin, an infection, stress and several other factors caused Katie to go into insulin shock. "I had an awful time," she said. "My sugar was 550 or higher and I was without my parents. I had trouble breathing, and I became dehydrated. I wound up having to spend three-and-a-half days in the hospital."

This incident forced Katie to withdraw from the competition, but it hasn't soured her on cheerleading; she's still an active member of her school's cheer squad.

Diabetes has not stopped her from doing the things she wants to do. Katie said, "I like to be real active in school with sports and academics.

"I don't think about the negatives of diabetes a lot; I play the piano and work out. I love hanging out with my friends. I don't let it bother me with my friends; we do pretty much what we want to do. We go out to eat all the time; I just watch my sugar and fat intake very closely."

Down the road, Katie wants to be a pharmacist. "Without the help of God, there's no way I could have gotten through the tough times," Katie said. "I've got tremendous parents (her father Danny and mother Judy) and a tremendous brother (Jay). My parents have encouraged me to be independent; my mom has always been very encouraging to me. She knows how to handle my diabetes, and I really admire her for that!"

CHAPTER 10

Getting Pumped

In the fight against diabetes, those suffering with the disease look for any edge they can possibly find.

Take Karen Boggs, a 29-year-old wife and mother from Westminster, S.C.

Attached to her body is a device that represents the latest in technology against diabetes – a pump that distributes insulin inside of her throughout the day.

Thanks to the pump, Boggs can escape the normal routine of shot after shot that those with diabetes in her situation usually have to go through.

Boggs gets insulin from the pump at 7 a.m., 10 a.m., noon, 3 p.m., 7 p.m. and throughout the night. Every hour, a small amount of insulin is distributed through the device, keeping her blood-sugar levels in a safe range. The only problem she has noticed with the pump is that it has left a small knot in her body. She has moved the needle to an area slightly above her navel, which has made it more comfortable for her.

"It's a wonderful device," Boggs said. "It gives you a lot of freedom, but I don't exercise much like I used to. It was very inconvenient for me exercising.

"I'm in a lot better control with the pump."

Boggs came down with diabetes when she was only 8 years old. "I had a virus," she recalled, "and I was at my grandmother's house. I kept eating old peppermint balls, and the more I ate, the sicker I got. My grandmother called my mother, and my mother called Dr. Julius Earle (a physician in the South Carolina Upstate)."

Earle detected her diabetes immediately, and she had to learn how to give herself injections quickly. Diabetes, though, didn't slow her down; she was a cheerleader in high school, and her parents used to bring a Glucagon kit with them to games when she was cheering.

"It was harder on them than it was on me when I participated in cheerleading and things like that," Boggs recalled.

She graduated in 1983 and married her sweetheart, Scott,

three years later. She was instructed by her doctors not to even think about having children, but she disregarded that and did get pregnant. During the pregnancy, she had to test her sugar 4-6 times per day and have four injections per day in order to stay healthy.

Her pregnancy was not smooth, and the child had to be delivered by Caesarean section at seven months. She said she had to do a lot of praying. "We prayed and prayed and prayed for her survival," Boggs said. "The prayers worked; my daughter, Brittany, was born and immediately taken to (a hospital in Greenville, S.C.). I hadn't held her or touched her when she was taken away.

"We prayed, called, prayed and called that she would be all right. I wanted God to know we wanted a child more than anything."

Even though she was a premature baby, Brittany is a healthy, happy, normal child. Today, she is 7 years old and the apple of her parent's eyes.

Karen believes that people with diabetes should seek expert medical attention to receive proper care. Two years ago, she went to Atlanta to see Dr. Chris Reed. "He's a wonderful doctor and person," she said. "He started me on carb counting. For example, if your sugar is at 160, you subtract 100 from it and divide by 30, and that's the amount of insulin I take for my sugar. They started me on four shots a day, treating the disease aggressively.

"Dr. Reed is a bit crazy, but he's down to earth. The first time I met him, he was blowing his nose, taking a mist spray and joking about it. One time, he came through where I live near Westminster and called just to see how I was feeling. That's the kind of doctor I want to go to."

Karen is an employee at U.S. Engine Valve, as is her husband. He has been a tremendous help in managing her diabetes and has always been there for her. Even her daughter will say to her sometimes, "Mom, don't you think you ought to take your blood sugar?"

Karen is glad she spent the $5,000 to give the pump a try. "It's really helped me a lot," she said.

CHAPTER 11

Like Father, Like Son

They say that diabetes tends to run in families.

You've already read about my cousin Mike and his battle with this disease, but I'd like to introduce you to Dr. Rob Lindemann and his son John.

Both of them have diabetes, Rob since he was 10 years old, while John has had it for some 18 months.

Despite the disease, Rob Lindemann has become one of the most respected internal medicine/diabetes physicians in Rock Hill, S.C., located near Charlotte.

"I had just gotten back from summer vacation when I developed diabetes," Rob recalled. "Statistically, it seems as if most people are diagnosed as diabetics in the spring or the fall.

"I was in the hospital for about a week when I was diagnosed. Before that, I was exhibiting all the classic symptoms. I was going to the bathroom all the time, for instance. I had to learn how to give myself shots and basically how to be a good diabetic."

He recalls having to use bulk glass syringes, the standard at the time. "They must have weighed about three pounds," Rob said. "The metal needles were boiled and reused over and over. I took one shot a day, and we never mixed insulin back then."

Despite his problems, Rob was very active in high school, playing golf and wrestling. He always knew while in high school that he wanted to go to medical school. "I always enjoyed school," Rob stated happily.

He eventually got his undergraduate degree and attended the Indiana University School of Medicine in Bloomington, Ind. He knew he wanted to be a part of treating those with diabetes and focused on learning about internal medicine. He knew many teens badly needed someone to talk to because he had dealt with the problems of diabetes at that young age himself.

Today, about 75 percent of his practice is geared toward people with diabetes. Eventually, he would like to see 100 percent of his practice devoted to people with diabetes and their unique problems. "I see this practice as an opportunity to help those with diabetes live normal, productive lives," Rob said. "It's important that diabetics get someone in close proximity to them who is very competent in diabetes."

Rob came to Rock Hill in 1980, following stints in Chapel Hill and Wilmington, N.C. His wife, Lori, is a nurse, and they have four children: Matt, 21; Paul, 16; John, 13; and Christine, 11.

It is the youngest son, John, who is very special to Rob and Lori, for, after all, John also has diabetes.

"It was devastating for me when I first learned John had diabetes," Rob recalled. "Having diabetes myself was one thing, but for him to have it was another thing altogether."

Rob has spent much time talking to his son about what to do for his diabetes and says John is doing just fine.

Diabetes is a challenge, Rob says. "You can control almost 100 percent of the potential complications if you do what you are supposed to do," he said.

To me, the medical profession needs more doctors who care about their patients like Dr. Rob Lindemann does and who are dedicated to help find a cure for diabetes.

Chapter 12

Red Cross and Empty Syringe

While diabetes in any form is a serious disease, not all people with diabetes have to take two, three or even four injections of insulin a day. Some watch what they eat and establish a routine that can become somewhat boring after awhile.

As most people with diabetes know, there are two types of diabetes – Type I, or insulin-dependent, and Type II, or non insulin-dependent.

Chicago-area native Roberta Nosko, who is the executive director of the Pickens County (S.C.) American Red Cross chapter, has Type II diabetes. In many respects, she feels very lucky to have escaped (at least for now) having to take injections and some of the other details those with Type I diabetes have to pay attention to.

Nosko developed her diabetes while pregnant with her second child, Michael. "I became fatigued and had good and bad days," Nosko said. "I started losing strength and felt very weak."

After a Glucometer test with her obstetrician, it was discovered she had gestational diabetes. "I felt fuzzy all the time," she said. "My blood sugar count was running 400 before they began injecting me with insulin.

"I guess thinking about the injections must have thrown me into shock. It had a very bad psychological effect on me."

Nosko feared she would be insulin-dependent for the rest of her life because of the gestational diabetes, but so far, she has been able to stay off insulin. Seven years after the fact, she is now controlling her diabetes through pills and diet.

She remains very busy, always on the go with her position with the Red Cross. But she hasn't forgotten what it's like to have diabetes.

"Diabetes is sneaky and insidious," she said. "Diabetes is not going to go away; it has to be treated right. You have to monitor your diet strictly and try to exercise. I'm stable right now and not even taking medicine, only controlling it through my diet. The doctor tells me, though, that eventually, it will change."

The mere thought of having to go on insulin is somewhat

frightening to Nosko. "I think about it every day, and it scares me," Nosko said.

She maintains a busy schedule, but she said that, without the help of a supportive staff, controlling her diabetes with diet only would be next to impossible. "I'm extra fortunate to have a great staff who are extra supportive," she said. "I can't stress enough that every person with a chronic illness needs to be around a group of people, a friend or a special person who can offer support. If I drop low, they'll tell me I need to eat something, for instance."

Nosko said having diabetes has taught her to respect other people who have chronic illnesses and made her realize that everyone is responsible for his or her own health.

CHAPTER 13

Voice of the Diabetic South

HOW SWEET IT IS

(Feasting On a Diabetic's Diet)

I will tell you a secret most quiet,
How to feast on a diabetic's diet.
Eat bread and eat meat,
But nothing that's sweet.
And never an egg, if you fry it.

Whenever you have some grave doubt
If it's good, you must spit it out;
Although you can deplore it,
You can never ignore it;
Too much good stuff gives you gout.

Eat peas, but leave off the cheese,
And honey created by bees.
Consume lots of greens,
Tomatoes and beans;
But pass up cake, if you please.

> Well, that's my advice, kindly take it,
> Remember to boil and to bake it.
> Frying it's bad,
> And sauteing is sad;
> But life is what you choose to make it.

Poems like these, as well as a humor column called *Kudzu Corner* that appears in the *Journal/Tribune* in Seneca, S.C., and *The Messenger* in Clemson, S.C., have kept Carroll Gambrell's many readers in Upstate South Carolina in stitches over the years.

He's even found time to write two well-accepted regional novels, *The Kudzu Chronicles* and *The Sugar Valley Saga*, both of which sold very well in South Carolina and throughout the Southeast.

Despite all that, however, it's a pretty safe bet not many of his readers know this about him:

Carroll Gambrell is a person with diabetes, having come down with it at age 38, a year following an operation to remove gallstones. "I remember thinking very strongly, when I was first diagnosed," he recalled, "that I had left one world and entered another one, one which I could not escape.

"No matter what I did, I would always be in this new world. I knew there would always be a barrier of separation between me and non-diabetics."

Gambrell first encountered the complications of diabetes when he noticed his vision was starting to deteriorate. "I went to the doctor back during the days when they had just developed throwaway syringes," Gambrell said. "They hadn't developed glucometers and machines for testing at home yet. They started me on Diabinase (a form of insulin) for about a year-and-a-half to control my diet.

"That came pretty naturally to me, thanks to my wife Ginger. She just happens to be a nurse."

It soon became apparent to Gambrell that his disease was going to force him to make many sacrifices in his lifestyle. "I quit thinking about things that were formerly very important to me, like an extra slice of chocolate cake," Gambrell said. "You can't pretend like you don't have diabetes. Your head might think it, but your body knows better."

Gambrell has encountered several instances where his sugar level dropped dangerously low, but Ginger always had hard candy around. He has had some close calls, including one in 1980 when, for two weeks, he was completely bedridden and his sugar level was over 600. "I smelled like a Dixie cup," Gambrell said. "Everything is sweet when you are in a situation like that; you have a sweet taste in your mouth.

"During this time, I began to see everyone in my life that ever meant anything to me. They would say a word or make a gesture. They made me feel so good. I knew at this point, dying would be easy. I also knew I had to take my insulin daily and do what I was supposed to do."

Gambrell spent several years in forestry work after obtaining a bachelor's degree in forestry from the University of Florida in Gainesville. But writing was something he always wanted to do, and once he retired from forestry work, he proceeded to go to work on his novels.

He didn't enjoy taking injections in the beginning, but even he admits he makes a pretty big target for the needle. His wife typically will give him the shot he needs each day.

Gambrell ultimately suffered a stroke, which is one of the potential complications of diabetes. He has no idea how much his diabetes played a role in it. The right side of his body was weakened by the stroke, and today, he walks with a limp. His face is somewhat crooked and his hands are not coordinated as they once were.

"Diabetes has caused me to live more of an orderly existence, which is good for me," he said. "Ginger is such a help for me. The fact that she is a nurse makes her aware of my needs and helps me deal with some of my problems."

Gambrell takes two injections each day and checks his levels twice a day. His wife makes sure the meals are properly fixed and are in front of him.

Diabetes has shown up in his family once again with the recent diagnosis of his brother Bob, aged 69. He hopes his son Forrest, 35, and daughter Erin, 30, won't have to struggle with diabetes. He also hopes for a future cure for the disease.

In the meantime, he'll write more columns and more novels. He probably will remain a favorite of people to talk to, thanks to his pleasant, easy-going manner.

We should all be so lucky to know a wonderful person like Carroll Gambrell.

CHAPTER 14

On the Legislative Front

Steve Smith has had, by most accounts, a very interesting career.

He has represented the savings industry to the South Carolina General Assembly in Columbia for more than 20 years, serving as president of the Community Financial Institutions of South Carolina organization since 1979 before announcing his resignation by Sept. 30, 1995, to establish a private consulting business.

Legislators in Columbia respect him. The community banks of the Palmetto State think he has been a godsend.

But Steve Smith also has had to battle many things in the 20 years he has been in Columbia.

One of the battles he wages daily is the battle against diabetes.

Smith has devoted much of his free time to the cause; in fact, he currently is the chair for the South Carolina Affiliate of the American Diabetes Association. As a person with diabetes, he has first-hand knowledge of the destruction diabetes does in South Carolina and throughout the nation.

Smith learned in 1989 that he had diabetes. One of the things that has bothered Smith greatly is the fact that he has not been able to keep his pilot's license because of his dependence on insulin; Federal Aviation Administration rules do not allow those with Type I diabetes to pilot aircraft.

Smith has learned to live with the illness, but having to give up his pilot's license still leaves him steamed. He plans to continue lobbying for a rules change that would allow those with diabetes in his situation to pilot planes.

"There would have to be a strict protocol set up, with quarterly tests and long-range tests conducted," Smith said. "Some very strict standards would have to be maintained. But there is no reason to deny someone a pilot's license, or take one away, just because he or she has to take insulin for this disease."

Smith came down with diabetes at age 39. "I remember my vision getting fuzzy," he recalled, "and I had an insatiable thirst and was constantly drinking water and fluids.

"Those two symptoms gave it away."

Smith immediately began treatment for his diabetes, first taking Micronase for his condition. "It got to the point where my weight had gone from 170 to 140 in just two years," Smith said. "I got to the point where I gave up the pills and let them put me on insulin.

"I felt better almost immediately."

Every day, Smith thanks God that insulin was developed in 1921 by two Canadian researchers, Drs. Frederick Banting and Charles Best. Without this medication, Smith knows that he would surely die of this disease.

He walks for 45 minutes each day on a treadmill and does situps and other exercises as part of the regimen he must follow. He takes three injections a day under an intense management regimen, adjusting his insulin depending on where his blood-sugar readings lie, which keeps him from extreme highs and lows.

Smith believes the best treatment for those who are insulin-dependent is the insulin pump. "I know people on it, and they swear by it," Smith said. "All you have to do is push a button, and you get insulin right away."

It's a good bet Smith will continue his lobbying to allow those with Type I diabetes to fly. But he will also keep up his work with the ADA on behalf of South Carolinians who have diabetes.

"I love working with the ADA," he said, "and exchanging information with different people. One of the things that has been beneficial for me is staying in contact with some of the top medical experts in their fields."

CHAPTER 15

The Feistiest Amputee

George Kuba is just a retiree who enjoys life.

But unlike many retirees in his community, Kuba, a native of Lake Zurich, Ill., near Chicago, is a person with diabetes – and a person who has lost a leg to the disease.

"I've been a person with diabetes for the past 27 years," Kuba explained. "I found out I had the disease when I underwent my yearly physical exam. I had to give a urine specimen as part of the exam, and when they tested it, they found it to be full of sugar.

"I went on oral medication at first and did all right on that for awhile, but one day, when I was serving on the Lake Zurich Board of Trustees, I went out with the other members and the mayor. I asked for a Diet Coke, but was served a regular Coke by mistake.

"That Coke was so full of sugar, I just about went into a diabetic coma. I had to be taken to the hospital and pumped full of insulin to get my level back to normal."

It was that experience that led Kuba to become insulin-dependent. Today, he injects himself twice a day, checks his blood sugar level three times a week and watches his diet very carefully, thanks to the efforts of his wife, Lori.

Kuba had been getting along well until one day when, as he was traveling to the Chicago area for his granddaughter's wedding and some Lions Club International business, something suddenly went wrong.

"I was having a really nice time, with many things to look forward to," Kuba said. "But that morning, at about 2 o'clock, something in my left leg closed up. I was in tremendous pain, I couldn't sleep and I had to get myself to a hospital right away."

Problem: The nearest hospital was three hours away, in Elgin, Ill.

When he did get there, he had to wait several more hours for X-rays to be taken – precious hours that, in fact, proved to be crucial.

"The X-rays showed the blockage in my leg, and it never

opened up again," Kuba recalled. "The doctors got together and decided they had to amputate my leg below the knee."

His first reaction to the decision was one of panic. "Here I was, a great athlete at Morton Township High School (now Morton East) in Cicero, Ill., a guy who ran a 4:20 mile in the late 1930s, and now, they were talking about cutting off my leg.

"Believe me, I wasn't particularly excited about that prospect."

Fortunately, Kuba had a very understanding doctor, and before the amputation was performed, he came in and explained to Kuba exactly what the operation would be like and his other options. "He explained everything they would do in an amputation, but he also explained what a vein graft might be like, and I decided to get the leg cut off," Kuba said.

While the operation was a relatively quick one, the sensation of it lasted much longer.

"They had me in the intensive care unit under heavy sedation," Kuba recalled. "The operation itself only lasted about three hours, but I think they wanted to get my mind off what had happened, which is why they kept me sedated."

The amputation and its aftermath caused Kuba to miss his granddaughter's wedding, but before they left on their honeymoon, the couple stopped by his hospital room and staged another ceremony for his benefit.

"That was really great of them to do that," he recalled. "My granddaughter wanted me to be a part of her wedding, and she went out of her way to come to my room and have another ceremony for me."

Life after his amputation wasn't the easiest. But for Kuba, it certainly was an adjustment he was willing to make.

"I knew that I had just had my leg cut off, but in my mind, I still had it," Kuba recalled. "One time while I was in the hospital, I woke up and had to go to the bathroom. Of course, this was very early in the morning, and my mind still told me I had my leg.

"Well, I got off the bed and started to walk to the restroom. Of course, I wound up falling right on the floor."

The crash brought nurses to his room, all of them somewhat upset.

"They asked me what I was doing not getting on my wheelchair, and I told them I couldn't remember my leg was gone," Kuba said. "Fortunately, they all had a sense of humor about it. They soon put a sign next to me reminding me that I had my leg amputated and to use the wheelchair next time!"

"Having to be fitted for an artificial leg was an aggravating process," Kuba recalled. "The first thing that happens is that they take a cast of your leg, then custom-fit a device for you. The first time I put it on, I screamed a lot; it didn't fit very well. They had to make several adjustments to get it to fit right.

"Eventually, your leg settles in and you have no more problems with the device. I had to learn how to walk with it, and they wanted me to use some crutches at first, saying that it would be about a year before I could walk normally again. I told them I didn't want to walk with crutches, and I learned quickly how to walk without it.

"It's something you certainly can't cry about. It happened, you accept it, adjust to it and move on with your life. One thing I want to show people is I'm not what can be called a *brittle* diabetic; I can do just about anything any normal person can do, and do it well. I have what's called a 'lazy pancreas'; it does produce insulin, but not enough to keep me well."

What kind of advice does Kuba have for people with diabetes?

"Simple," he said. "Be sure you know what the warning signs are and go to the doctor if you think you might have it.

There's not a cure for diabetes *yet*, so you have to really watch yourself and don't cheat on anything. If you cheat on anything, you're only cheating yourself.

"Just do what the doctor says and you'll be all right. It's a disease you don't have to let control you. You can certainly control *it*."

CHAPTER 16

"Diabetes is Sneaky"

The complications of diabetes can sometimes be dire.

Persons afflicted with this disease can lose a lot of things precious to them – their limbs, their ability to get around, their lifestyle.

Nothing can be more devastating, though, than for a person with diabetes to lose his or her eyesight because of the complications of the disease.

Just ask Hedwig Cliffe of Westminster, S.C.

The complications caused by diabetes cost Cliffe her eyesight and may wind up shortening her life.

Her blindness has only come on recently (as this chapter was being written in July 1995, she had only been declared legally blind over the past six months). But once the eye problems took hold, they progressed very quickly.

"All I can see now are shadows of objects," Cliffe, a native of Stuttgart, Germany, said. "I used to have very good eyesight, but because of the disease, it really deteriorated.

"It has been very hard on me and my husband. I cannot do the things I used to be able to do, like cleaning and cooking."

Hedwig's blindness has forced her husband, James, to take over most of the household duties Hedwig did.

"I certainly can do them, but I had to quit my job (he had been working as a security guard) in order to help care for her," James said. "It's absolutely devastating. I believe in the marriage vows I took when I married her, and caring for her is something I am absolutely willing to do. But it's very, very difficult."

This experience has been both financially and emotionally draining for the Cliffes, and it has led them to believe one thing about diabetes:

"It's a sneaky, sneaky disease," James said. "It can devastate a person and his or her family, and many times, people don't even realize it's happening."

"When I first got diabetes," Hedwig added, "(the doctor) told me everything that could possibly happen to me as a diabetic, like going blind, going into congestive heart failure and the other complications associated with the disease.

"Everything he has said has come true."

Both of the Cliffes admitted to much ignorance of the disease before Hedwig came down with it. "I admit it, I was ignorant," Hedwig said. "I thought it wouldn't happen to me, that I would be the person who was the exception to the rule.

"I've learned that it could happen to me. I blame no one but myself for that."

When Hedwig first came down with diabetes in 1984, she took glucose pills in order to control the disease. She eventually had to begin injecting herself with insulin, but when blindness struck, she had to return to the pill routine, a routine that has proven to be very expensive.

"Our medical bills are more than $700 a month," James said, "yet our Medicare won't cover it. I pay $96 per month for Medicare and $101 for a supplement, and I only get $654 a month in Social Security benefits.

"You wonder what has happened in this country, especially to seniors. We're the forgotten Americans. We can spend some money on research to find a cure for cancer, but we hardly allocate any money at all for diabetes research. We need to have some legislation that addresses the needs of diabetics in this country. People with diabetes need help very badly. It's a horrible disease, yet hardly anyone devotes any time to it in this country."

Despite the hardships, Hedwig's ordeal has helped the couple grow much stronger than they ever thought possible. "It's been rough," James said, "but despite it, we've also grown closer together than ever. I believe a husband should help his wife as much as possible in a case like this.

"The Lord's helped us so far; He's been a source of a lot of grace to us. I don't know what we would do without His help."

For those who are newly diagnosed persons with diabetes, the Cliffes have some simple advice:

"If you feel sick, go to the doctor as soon as you can," Hedwig said. "Please listen to what he has to say and follow his orders exactly. That's the only way anyone can win against this horrible disease."

"It's a dangerous and sneaky disease," James added. "I hope anyone who reads this, especially a young person, won't dismiss this as some sort of hogwash. It can happen to anyone, and can strike anytime.

"It'll hit you hard and just when you least expect it."

CHAPTER 17

You Can't Give Up

Losing one leg to diabetes is bad enough.

Losing both legs can be devastating.

But despite losing both of her legs to this disease, Willa Bailey, a 75-year-old black woman, hasn't gotten down about it.

"It's not as tough and difficult as someone might think," Bailey said. "It hasn't been the easiest thing in the world, but you can't complain about it. You just have to move on and adapt to everything the best you can."

Bailey lost her legs 11 years apart, her left leg in 1984 and her right leg in 1995. Both times, the complications of diabetes were to blame.

How she learned she had the disease was perhaps typical of many with diabetes, who often can have the disease for years and not even realize it.

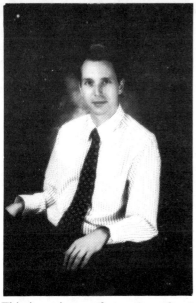

This is a picture of me taken after I had contracted diabetes, but before I began taking insulin. As you can see, I looked like I was just waiting for good breeze to knock me down!

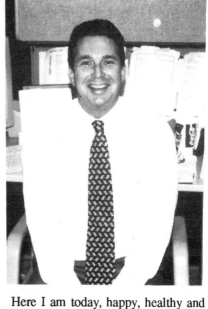

Here I am today, happy, healthy and leading a fairly normal life. If insulin hadn't been discovered, it's a good bet I wouldn't even be writing this book right now. I owe my life to insulin.

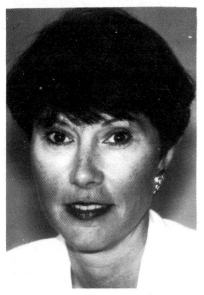

This is Cindy Floyd, my diabetes educator in Seneca, S.C. Cindy has been a very valuable source of information for me in my fight against the disease.

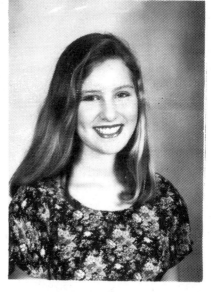

Katie Plemmons has it all — looks, brains, determination — and Type I diabetes. Since she came down with the disease, Katie has been very outspoken about diabetes.

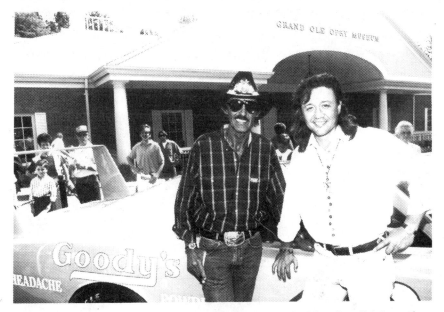

Mark Collie is a well-known country music star — and has insulin-dependent diabetes. He established the Mark Collie Celebrity Race for Diabetes Cure in Nashville in 1994 and got the King of NASCAR — Richard Petty — to be the grand marshal for the inaugural race. The two-day event turned out to be a huge success.

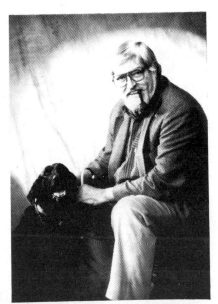

Carroll Gambrell is a well-known Southern humorist, author — and a long-term person with diabetes. "You enter another world when you get diabetes," he says.

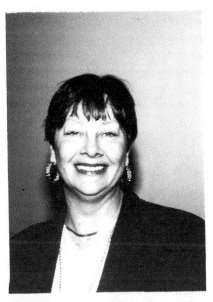

Roberta Nosko is a Red Cross director in Pickens, S.C., and has Type II diabetes. While not as severe as Type I diabetes, Type IIs still need to watch themselves.

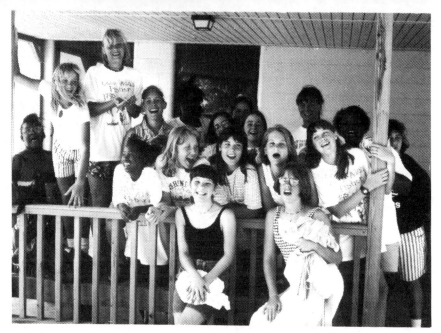

Camp Adam Fisher, located near Summerville, S.C., is one of the nation's oldest summer camps for children with diabetes. It has often been described as the happiest place in South Carolina — and these obviously happy campers are eager to show it!

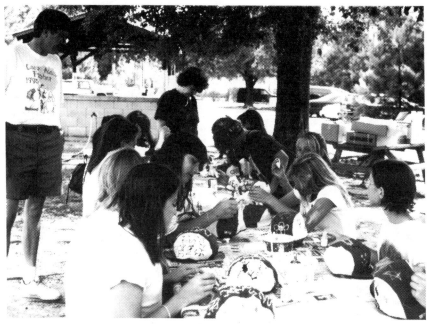

Arts and crafts are a traditional part of any summer camp, even Camp Adam Fisher in South Carolina, as these campers show. Not only do the campers take home their creations, they take home some wonderful memories, too.

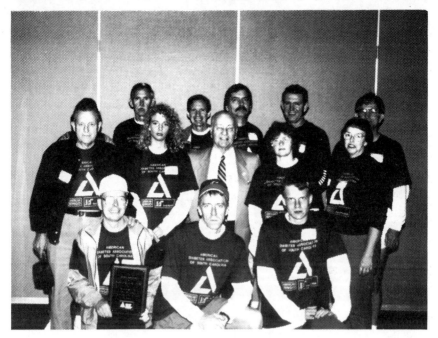

Every Thanksgiving weekend, a dedicated group of runners gathers together in South Carolina for the annual Turkey Trot Mountains to the Sea run for diabetes. The run starts in the mountains by the Georgia-South Carolina border and ends three days later at the world-famous resort town of Myrtle Beach. The run has raised thousands of dollars over the years.

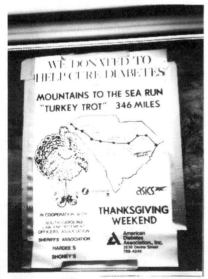

As you can see, the Mountains to the Sea run covers a good portion of Palmetto real estate — nearly 350 miles worth, in fact.

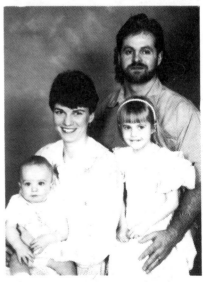

Here is the inspiration for the Mountains to the Sea Run — Sherri Morrison, her husband, Roger and their children Graysen and Camden.

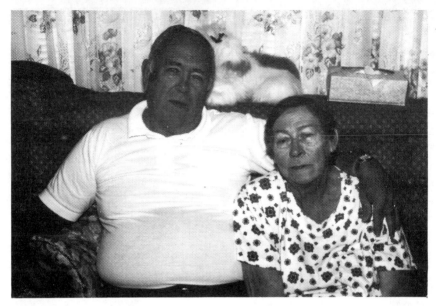

James and Hedwig Cliffe are a typical South Carolina couple, except in one sense—Hedwig has gone blind because of diabetes. Blindness is one of the major complications of this disease, one that costs the American economy millions each year. Yet not nearly enough money is being allocated to find a cure for this disease.

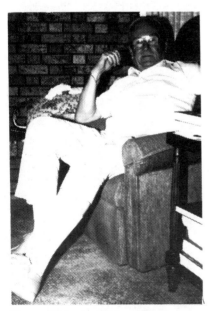

George Kuba is a Chicagoland native who lost a leg to diabetes. Yet the loss of his leg hasn't dulled his working-class spirit— or his sense of humor.

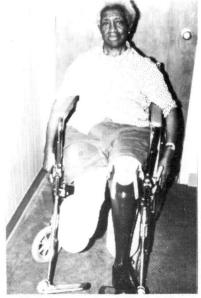

Willa Bailey has lost both her legs to diabetes. When the second leg had to come off, her family protested, but her faith in God has helped her.

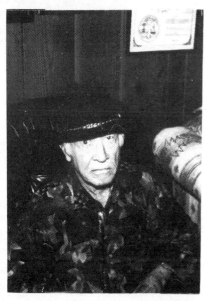

Daniel Land is simply known as D. to his friends. He's been a champion dancer, cowboy, actor — and has had diabetes since 1963. Despite nearing 90, diabetes hasn't slowed him.

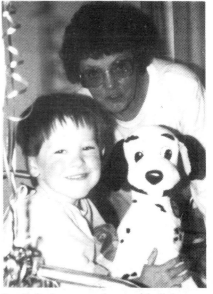

Justin Stokes came down with diabetes at a very early age. He's learned to work with, but not accept, his disease. His parents have formed a support group in South Carolina for children with diabetes.

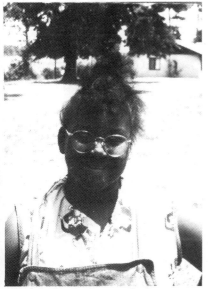

Kristen Jacobs is a typical pre-teen girl — and has Type I diabetes. Kristen is one of the many kids who attend Camp Adam Fisher each year in Summerville, S.C., on property owned by Clemson University.

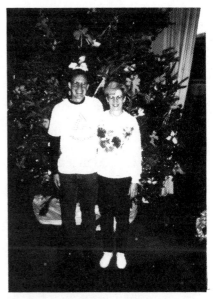

Maurice and Marlene Poore are the parents of Sherri Morrison — the inspiration and driving force behind the annual Mountains-to-the-Sea run.

"I have been a diagnosed person with diabetes since 1970," Bailey recalled when she was interviewed in the health-care home where she currently resides. "My sister, Lois Lewis, was also a person with diabetes, so it runs in both sides of our family. Anyway, I was living in Greenville, S.C., and working in a hotel kitchen there. One morning, I got up feeling well and went to work that day. All of a sudden, I felt very sick and weak. I sent for the chef, and he took one look at me and sent me to a doctor he knew.

"The doctor took one look at me and kept me at his office for a very long time. No one told me right away what was wrong. Then, the nurse came in and ran a test on me, then took a blood sample. The doctor looked at it and told me I was a person with diabetes and my blood sugar level was high enough for me to go into a diabetic coma.

"The first thing the doctor told me was that I had to get my weight down. At that time, I weighed 226 pounds, so I started pushing the plate away from me at mealtimes. It wasn't easy, but I did it."

The diet reduced her weight and had other positive side effects, one of which was seeing her dress size going from size 16 to size 14.

Several years later, Bailey's diabetes worsened to the point where she had to learn how to give herself injections, a frightening prospect for anyone scared by even the thought of needles.

Not Bailey.

"I never was frightened by the needle," she said. "It was something I just had to learn how to do, and I managed to do it pretty well."

In 1984, Bailey began to notice something was wrong with her left heel. She told her doctor about it. "I kept telling the doctor there was something wrong with my heel, and he X-rayed it and shot me in the hip," Bailey recalled. "He kept saying I was all right, but one morning, I tried to put a bedroom shoe on, and I couldn't even stand to do that. The doctor took another look, gave me a pain shot and said I was all right."

But Bailey knew something was terribly amiss.

"One morning, a nurse who was visiting me sent me to bed and told me to stay there," Bailey said. "The next day, I went to see Dr. David Irvine. He looked at me and sent me to the nursing department at Clemson University.

"The nurses there looked at me and told me, 'Honey, you got some problems.' "

A hole had eaten through Bailey's heel. Irvine trimmed the dead flesh and infection from her heel and sent her to the hospital for therapy, which included whirlpool sessions. When that didn't work, she was sent to another hospital for treatment and therapy.

Two doctors examined her leg and realized this treatment wasn't enough.

"After some time, the doctor came in to talk to me and told me they had done everything they could to save the leg, and it looked as though they were going to have to amputate it, but they wanted to talk to me about it first before doing anything. They asked me what I thought about it, and I agreed that it would be for the best."

Eleven years later, Bailey started experiencing problems with her right leg. "I had been having trouble sleeping, just tossing and turning," Bailey said. "My leg was really bothering me and my foot was starting to hurt.

"There were sores on my foot that eventually burst open and became ulcerated. The doctor took one look at me and told me I was going to the hospital right away.

"They ran tests, even put some sort of dye in my leg to see what was wrong. Finally, they had no choice. They had to amputate the other leg."

Losing the other leg created a crisis in her family. "One of my nieces asked me how was I going to walk again, and I told her, 'With God's help, I can walk.' It wasn't anything I was looking forward to having done to me, but it was something I had to do.

"I cried when the other leg was taken off; I didn't want it to happen. But I saw a thing on television where kids without any legs were playing ball, and I thought to myself, 'If they can stand it, so can I.' "

Bailey today has prostethic devices she uses to get around, one she has had since her left leg was amputated, the other one she was just learning how to use at the time this was written.

"It's not been easy, but you can't complain too much," Bailey said. "If nothing else, I'm still here, and that's a lot more than what some other people can say."

CHAPTER 18

The Diabetic Cowboy

Daniel Land has done just about everything a person can imagine.

He's been a cowboy. A dancer. A bullrider. A mason. Even a stuntman and actor in films, including a 1955 Walt Disney film, *The Great Locomotive Chase.*

In his 88 years, Land – known simply as D. to his friends – has done it all.

Since 1963, everything Land has done has been with a certain condition in mind – diabetes.

He's not exactly in the best of health these days; a severe heart attack suffered in 1994 slowed him down considerably. But his life remains an interesting one.

"I had always been very active," Land said. "During my younger adult years, you know, I was a cowboy. I went to a lot of rodeos and took part in them; I even took part in the Frontier Days Rodeo in Cheyenne, Wyo., one year.

"They wouldn't let me ride when I was there (because, Land said, he had no membership in what is now known as the Professional Rodeo Cowboys Association). I really wanted to get into the bull riding contest. I stayed after them and finally, they let me into the event. I wound up riding a couple of bulls, and I did pretty well. Even made (a mention in) *The Denver Post*."

Land and his wife, after returning to the South Carolina Upstate, built a western-style town behind his home in Seneca. They erected an old country church, blacksmith shop and other items.

The small town they built turned into a major attraction.

"It took me about 25 years (to build everything in the town)," Land told *Foxfire*, a high school magazine in Georgia (the source of some of the information in this profile). "All of the buildings took me about 25 years. I mean, I made them; nobody helped me.

"On Easter, we have sunrise service up (at the church) at 7 o'clock...we had 65 weddings in there. It tied us up all the time. We couldn't do anything. Every time we wanted to go somewhere, Bessie (his wife) said, 'We can't go. We got a wedding coming up.'"

Land developed his diabetes back in 1963, a time when treatments were more advanced than they had been 30 years earlier, but nowhere near as advanced as they are today.

"I had been feeling pretty dizzy," Land recalled, "and not feeling well. I decided to go to the doctor, and he sent me to Anderson for some tests. When they came back, they showed that I had diabetes."

Despite that diagnosis, Land, who had always been a very active person, refused to take it lying down.

"I was a boxer in my younger days; even fought in some amateur tournaments (as a welterweight)," Land recalled. "I did pretty well, but I really had no killer instinct. I went into the ring wanting to do well enough to win. I never wanted to hurt my opponent."

The boxing habits Land picked up during his fighting days have served him well in his battle against diabetes. "Even today, I have a heavy bag that I'll work on for exercise," he said. "It's really helped me out very well. I'll go in there and hit it for awhile to keep in pretty good shape."

Land was very lucky; he was able to control his condition with tablets and exercise until 1985, when he finally had to start injecting himself with insulin.

"I inject myself with 38 units of insulin each morning when I wake up, then test my blood sugars during the day," Land said about his daily routine. "If my level is at 300 or more, then I'll inject myself with 15 more units at about 2 p.m.

"Fortunately, that second injection doesn't happen too often. Being as active as I've been, I've been able to keep my levels pretty normal."

Land is living proof that having diabetes doesn't force a person, regardless of age, to live an inactive lifestyle.

"I've never had too many problems with diabetes," Land said. "Anyone with diabetes can feel good and feel normal. All you have to do is take care of yourself and don't let it run your life.

"I've got no worries about having diabetes. It's just the way it is. If you do what you have to do and follow your doctor's advice, you'll be just fine. You don't have to become a slave to this disease. You can control it; it doesn't have to control you."

CHAPTER 19

She's The Inspiration

═══════════

In the movie *Steel Magnolias*, the character Shelby dies after giving birth to her first child. Shelby, played by Julia Roberts, was a person with diabetes who was urged not to have children, but did so anyway.

Sherri Morrison has been a person with diabetes since she was 9 years old and always understood the dangers of someone with her illness having a child. Originally, she never planned on having children and had made a decision to try to adopt a child with her husband, Roger.

But being the optimists both are, the couple soon decided they would not adopt, but attempt to have a child of their own.

Sherri became pregnant while her husband was stationed in Hawaii with the U.S. Navy. She had to increase her insulin shots to three a day and test her blood sugar eight times a day.

"I had to set an alarm clock at 2 each morning to test my sugar," said Sherri. "I had to call my doctor, Ursula Heinz, every day. She was a German doctor and I can remember her constantly saying, 'Sherri, this is very bad' in her German accent."

Sherri and Roger waited until Christmas 1989 to inform her parents, Maurice and Marlene Poore, of their decision to have a child.

Marlene cried and cried after she learned Sherri was pregnant.

"I felt so awful about it at the time," said Marlene.

Sherri continued her care with Dr. Heinz through the entire process. Without Dr. Heinz's constant attention, it is doubtful Sherri's pregnancy would have gone nearly as well.

Sherri was due Aug. 2, 1990, but her first baby, Cambren, was born on July 8, 1990, by Caesarean section.

"Dr. Heinz told me I should enjoy Cambren," said Sherri. "She told me I was lucky how things turned out. I was so happy. I never thought I'd have a child because of the diabetes and all the things I'd been told."

Sherri learned a great deal having the first baby and thought she was capable of having another one.

Sherri and Roger's second child, Graysen, was born nearly three years later.

The second pregnancy was much easier, Sherri said.

"I guess I knew what to expect," she said. "My doctor, Perry DeLoach in Clemson, S.C., wasn't quite as regimented. He expected and required his patients to take an active role in their health care.

"He gave me a formula to adjust my insulin. He told me how much regular insulin to give and the other things to do. It was a pretty uneventful pregnancy. My son was born on schedule by Caesarean. Everything went as planned."

Today, Cambren, 5, and Graysen, 2, are as healthy as can be. Sherri, Robert, Marlene and Maurice, of course, wouldn't trade the way things are for anything in the world.

Sherri feels most fortunate to have her two wonderful children.

"I was told by doctors after I had the first child that I should feel fortunate," said Sherri. "The doctors told me to have one healthy child. And it was more important for my daughter to have a mother than for me to have another child."

Roger describes himself as an eternal optimist in life. He says life is too short to worry about things that can go wrong.

"I am so thankful for what I have," said Roger. "Sherri does a wonderful job being a wife and mother. I have really high expectations and I expect things to go well. I am very goal-oriented. Having a wife who has diabetes is challenging.

"The whole day has two pivotal points because she has to take her shots on schedule. It's a part of our daily routine. You take a shower, brush your hair and get a shot."

Sherri had an uneventful life until she was 9 years old, when her weight dropped to 63 pounds and neither father nor mother could figure out what was wrong with her.

"I didn't know exactly what was wrong with her," said her father. "The only thing we could refer to was a medical encyclopedia. One time, we were going to Greenville (S.C.) on a Saturday, and she starting crying. She had to go to the bathroom.

"The next week, she had wet the bed, and we knew something was seriously wrong. We also noticed her going to the sink to get water several times. We called the doctor and made an appointment. The doctor immediately diagnosed her as being a person with diabetes. We had no idea what was involved."

Sherri remembers her diagnosis, but didn't know exactly what was involved.

"I resented it a whole lot growing up," she said. "I hated to be singled out and looked at as being different. I was the only one in my whole school who had to take insulin.

"When I was younger, all the other kids would have chocolate milk, and when it came time for me to place my order, I had to get regular milk. I couldn't believe I was cursed like I was. I couldn't spend the night with other kids because I had to have a shot each morning. It was probably three or four years before I had the courage to give myself a shot. My parents worked with me a lot on my diet. Everything I ate was measured until I was a teen-ager. I never had any type of insulin reaction while I was growing up because my parents took such good care of me."

Marlene said Sherri had a hard time dealing with being a teen-ager with diabetes emotionally. Maurice always encouraged Sherri, though, with her exercise, which she detested. Her father would wake her up in the mornings and run with her a half-mile out and a half-mile back. The morning runs, ironically, laid the foundation for the Oconee Road Runners Club and, later on, the Thanksgiving weekend Run from the Mountains to the Sea, an annual fund-raiser for the South Carolina American Diabetes Association, which will be examined later on in this book.

"I still appreciate everything my parents did for me growing up," Sherri said.

At first, Roger never knew that Sherri was a person with diabetes when they met while both were attending Walhalla High School in South Carolina.

"I asked her if she wanted an ice cream, and she bluntly said 'No'," Roger recalled, "but she never told me at that time that she was a person with diabetes and couldn't have any. Eventually, she did tell me about her condition."

It's doubtful Sherri has forgotten all the broccoli, green peas and V-8 vegetable juice that was served at her house. It's certain she hasn't forgotten her father, who woke up with her each morning to run with her and keep her blood sugar levels down. Sherri's organs have been checked out and they are still in fantastic shape, despite having diabetes for more than 20 years.

Sherri said, "For those who want to do the right things, diabetes is controllable."

CHAPTER 20

Don't Stop Believing

Ricky Kimbrell hasn't had an easy life.

Ricky, who is 38, has been a person with diabetes since he was 10 years old.

The Seneca, S.C., man has already had a kidney transplant, a stroke, laser surgery on his eyes and other complications because of diabetes. But he hasn't let such setbacks sour his attitude on diabetes or his life.

Ricky remembered when he was first told he had diabetes. "I can remember the process of getting sick," he said. "I was so sick, I lost a lot of weight before I was carried to the hospital. They did the blood work, and then they called home and told everyone I had diabetes. I was in the hospital for about two weeks."

His sister Betty helped him with the shots he needed when Ricky couldn't do it himself, but growing up wasn't particularly easy. He couldn't go out and do the things other children his age could do.

"I felt kind of cheated and left out," he recalled. "I couldn't play football and the other things kids ordinarily did. I felt cheated; my teen-age years were pretty rough.

"I think diabetes held me back in school, as well. I was sick a lot."

After leaving high school, he went to Wendy's to work, then to Pratt Industries in Seneca, running a band saw for about 13 years.

His eyes were the first organ to deteriorate, about 10 years ago. Two years ago, his kidneys both failed pretty much at once; he had a transplant performed on March 6, 1994. He has had laser surgery on his eyes four times in an effort to save his sight.

The stroke he had took place in May 1995. As strokes go, it was pretty mild, and today, Ricky is doing well. But his health hasn't always been the best. Today, his weight is about 120 pounds. He has weighed about 145 in the past.

Ricky's sister, Betty Stancil, says it has been hard to deal with having to watch her brother suffer.

"My brother has always smiled and had a good attitude, despite all of his problems," Betty said. "Even when I took him to the hospital when he was having his stroke, he forced a smile on his face and told me he was going to be all right.

"Despite all that, it's been very difficult seeing him suffer like he has. I wish he hadn't had to go through what he has experienced in his life."

Ricky certainly urges people with diabetes to live life to the fullest and do whatever they want within the confines of the disease. "You can't go out the door with someone telling you what to do," he said.

Like many persons with diabetes, Ricky certainly hopes there will be a cure for the disease in the near future. "Diabetes has been kept under the covers for many years," Ricky said. "I'm glad to see so many people starting to talk about it today.

"I can see how I would have done a lot better if I had known all the things they know now about how to treat diabetes. But anyone with diabetes will tell you that you have to live life to the fullest and take things as they come."

CHAPTER 21

A Special Place for Kids

Nestled among the pine and the palmetto trees in the Lowcountry of South Carolina is a very special place for children with diabetes.

A place where, for one week during each summer, those children can get away from the daily problems they face with their disease and be like the average, everyday kid.

A place where they can swim, make crafts, meet tough challenges and gain the confidence that, despite having diabetes, they can take on the world - and win.

It's called Camp Adam Fisher, and it takes place at Clemson University's 4-H campsite, Camp Bob Cooper, on the shores of Lake Marion near the town of Sumter, S.C., approximately 50 miles from Charleston.

In many ways, the site looks like a typical summer camp.

On either side of the facility are dormitories that house campers who flock here from all over South Carolina and even a few from out-of-state. Nearby is a lake where swimming, boating and other water activities take place, while several nature trails, a challenge course and softball and football fields are on the other side.

In other words, Camp Bob Cooper is typical of what some people may think when they hear the words "summer camp."

Unlike the typical summer camp, though, Camp Adam Fisher is a week-long gathering of kids who don't dwell on the fact that they are children with diabetes.

"Camp Adam Fisher got started back in 1967," said Dr. Frank Bowyer, a pediatric endocrinologist at the University of South Carolina Medical School in Columbia and medical director for the camp. "It was started by a Greenville (S.C.) businessman named Adam Fisher who had a daughter who had contracted diabetes. He wanted his daughter to have the experience of attending a summer camp, but there were no camps in the region that could help her.

"He felt that his daughter should be able to go to a camp, so he raised some money with some other businessmen he knew and held his first camp for diabetic children in 1967 in Greenville.

Originally, it was known as Camp Did You Do It, as in 'did you take your insulin?,' for instance. As the camp grew and became so well-known and the contributions he made to the growth of the camp were so enormous, it was renamed in his honor."

The camp was run by Fisher until several years ago, when the American Diabetes Association's South Carolina chapter took it over. The camp has moved several times until it reached its current location in the Lowcountry, where today, anywhere between 100-130 children with diabetes aged 7-17 flock to the site for a week each summer of experiences that may have been previously denied them. In fact, Fisher, who is retired and living with his wife in an Inman, S.C., retirement home, attended the camp regularly until very recently.

"Adam still wants to know everything that goes on," said Cliff Moore, Youth Services Director for the ADA-SC and the man who has served as the camp's director. "Even though he can't make it here any more, he still has a great interest in the camp and what these kids are doing.

"Every year, when I get back from camp, I call Adam right away and let him know what happened during the week."

The Camp Bob Cooper facilities are an ideal place for Camp

Adam Fisher. "Camp Bob Cooper's facilities are about the biggest in the state, and we've really had a great working relationship with Clemson University over the years," Bowyer said. "They've bent over backwards to accommodate us and help us. They've helped us in every way possible. I don't think this camp would be possible without the generosity they've shown us over the years."

Not only does the camp benefit from CU's generosity, but the camp also has some very good friends throughout the state. "We have a very diverse group of people who have helped us over the years," Bowyer said. "We've had Shriners help us, members of the Eastern Star and other related organizations, even a Harley Owner's Group (or HOGs, as they are affectionately known by motorcycle enthusiasts everywhere) have pitched in to help the camp. Our kids sell coupon books and take part in other fund-raising activities, as well, to help out."

What is notable about Camp Adam Fisher is the fact that no child with diabetes is turned away because of a lack of finances. "We have scholarship-type financial aid that we give to our campers to help them come to camp and enjoy themselves," Bowyer said. "We have never turned a child away from camp just because his or her parents couldn't afford the cost."

And the kids, to say the least, are the most important part of this camp.

"To see these kids come back year after year, either as campers or even as counselors, and to see their faces light up, well, that's the best part about the whole thing," Moore said. "They're the future of this camp and of making diabetes known throughout the state and nation.

"Whenever they're in school or church, say, they may be the only one there who has diabetes. In that way, they are the unusual one. Here, they're surrounded by other kids from the state who have the same thing. They're not the unusual one. At Camp Adam Fisher, they can come here, be around other kids who have the same problems as they do and not feel strange."

Like most camps, Camp Adam Fisher has the same activities as other camps. "We have two (program) tracks here," Bowyer said. "One track is designed mostly for younger children and gives them the same activities as you might find at other camps."

"During the day, we offer activities such as swimming, horseback riding, arts and crafts, canoeing, paddleboat riding and free time where they can play football, basketball, softball, capture the flag and everything else. At night, we have dances, talent shows, carnival-type activities and a nightly campfire and vespers."

Another track is designed for older children and helps to build up the confidence of these children while giving them a sense of high adventure. "Our adventure track contains things like overnight campouts, a team course, tubing, sailing and even a challenge course that contains a 40-foot wall the kids attempt to scale (all while wearing a required safety harness)," Bowyer said. "One camper we had this year took on a 20-foot wall on one of the challenge courses and told me, 'If I can do this, I can do anything.'

"That's the whole idea behind these courses, to give our campers the confidence to take on the challenges of life they have to face and to help them realize that, even though they have diabetes, they're really no different from other kids."

A medical staff is always on duty to help campers should they run into trouble with injuries or if their blood-sugar level plunges too low. "We also schedule snacks and other meals with the kids and their condition in mind," Bowyer said. "We help them check their sugar levels and help them administer their daily insulin injections. We've got it to the point now where it flows really smoothly."

The bottom line at Camp Adam Fisher is a simple one: Just because they have diabetes doesn't mean children have to feel different.

"The message we have here at Camp Adam Fisher is that you can manage your disease and still be very happy," Bowyer said. "The friendships they form, the role models they meet, the bonding that takes place between each other is amazing. I mean, this is a very magical place."

"Just because they have diabetes doesn't mean they can't do the same things as normal kids," Moore added. "The only thing they can't do is eat a cake or drink a regular soda or have a candy bar.

"I wish people from all over the state could come here and see what goes on at Camp Adam Fisher. They would be amazed at what these special kids can do, despite the fact they are battling a very serious disease. I really think for one week every year, this is one of the happiest places in all of South Carolina."

Few would argue with that sentiment, especially those who have been involved in the camp or who have attended it. Just ask the counselors who have been a part of the camp over the years, especially those who have attended as campers and then as counselors.

"I grew up with the camp," said Paul Kinlaw, a 17-year-old

counselor from Goose Creek, S.C., who attended the camp for the previous eight years as a participant. "Being a camper was a lot of fun," Kinlaw said. "But there's a big difference between attending the camp as a camper and being a counselor at the camp. There's a lot more responsibility. Instead of being responsible for just yourself, you are responsible for other kids, as well.

"I've got 13-year-olds this year, and they're a handful. There are times when they just don't want to listen to you. But they're all good kids; all of them are really neat persons."

That's not to say that every day is fun and games. "The first night we were here, I had a camper nearly pass out on me," Kinlaw said. "I was running back and forth, trying to figure out what to do, and the kids knew what to do better than I did."

Another camp counselor, Kel Jansen, was diagnosed with diabetes only last year. "Getting diabetes has been a huge challenge for me," said the Columbia resident and University of South Carolina occupational therapy student. "I was hoping to go into the FBI, but after I got diabetes, I had to change my goals because of some regulations about people with the disease.

"It was a big disappointment for me. I couldn't figure out why I even came down with diabetes, but these days, I figure that

God wouldn't let me become a diabetic if he didn't think I could handle it."

Being a Camp Adam Fisher counselor was an eye-opening experience for Jansen. "I never knew anything about diabetes before I got it," Jansen said. "I came to Camp Adam Fisher four weeks after I learned I had the disease. The kids really taught me a lot about the disease, especially how to deal with living with it and accepting it as a normal part of life.

"I know it sounds unusual, but I learned as much from my kids about diabetes and how to handle it as from any other source. The kids here have lived with it for a number of years; I'll go as far as to say that they've all been a huge inspiration for me."

Why did Jansen decide to become a counselor? "I wanted to give something back, and I thought this would be a good way to do it," Jansen said. "If I can see a kid living with diabetes and not complaining about it, the least I can do is the same thing. They push me and challenge me to be my best; I can't say enough about how they've inspired me."

For those who come to Camp Adam Fisher as campers and stay on as counselors, the experiences and the friendships that develop are the reasons they keep coming back year after year.

"I've been here for the past 10 years," said Lugoff, S.C., native Vernon Tucker. "The people you meet here are the people you really care about. They're like sisters and brothers to me. We all share a lot of common experiences with diabetes."

Tucker admitted that, when he first came to camp, he was somewhat of a wild child. "I was so immature a camper at first," Tucker said. "I was worse than the devil himself. But after I had been gone awhile, I began to figure things out.

"When you come to this camp, the counselors and the leaders understand your problems, and you leave here knowing you're no different than anyone else who has diabetes.

"I can't say enough good things about this camp; it's been one of the best experiences of my entire life."

CHAPTER 22

The Faces of Adam Fisher

The approximately 100-130 participants in the American Diabetes Association-South Carolina's annual Camp Adam Fisher are as diverse a group as any in South Carolina.

They come from all sorts of families – the well-off, the middle-class, the poor, the struggling. They come from every ethnic background and religion. They range in age from 7-17. They have had many experiences in life, some good and some not good.

Despite all the differences, they have things in common: All of them have diabetes. They must inject themselves with insulin at various times of the day in order to survive. They risk their health if they ingest a sugary snack.

And one more thing:

All of them have hopes and dreams for their future.

Here are profiles of six of the 1995 Camp Adam Fisher participants. Each of them is a unique individual. Each of them has diabetes.

Their stories, their hopes, their dreams, are an inspiration to everyone:

Ashley Avinger
Age 11, Orangeburg, S.C.
Has attended Camp Adam Fisher for the past five years:

When Ashley Avinger found out she was a child with diabetes at age 6, her world seemed to cave in on her.

"I had no idea what diabetes was," the blond-haired youth recalled, her steel-blue eyes piercing right through any possible defenses. "I was just 6 years old, and I was pretty scared about what diabetes was.

"I thought everything in my life was going to go wrong from that point on. Everyone in my family was devastated."

Her condition was severe enough to the point where she had to start injecting herself just a few months later. It doesn't bother her now, though she does admit, with a bit of trepidation, "Having to give yourself shots can be scary. But you eventually get used to it, and now, it really doesn't bother me."

Her friends at school and in the neighborhood don't treat her any differently than others. "My friends understand my disease, but there are times when I can't eat certain things, and I feel a bit left out. There's really not a lot I can do about it."

When she grows up and finishes school, Ashley would like to be a doctor, perhaps going into general surgery. "My disease didn't inspire me to want to be a surgeon," she said. "It's just something I want to do with my life because I think it would be a great thing to do."

Kristen Jacobs
Age 12, Columbia, S.C.
Attended Camp Adam Fisher for the first time in 1995:

Attending Camp Adam Fisher was a new experience for Kristen, something she enjoyed but also found, surprisingly, a bit boring.

"A lot of it depends on the time of the day, but for the most part, I've had a lot of fun here," the dark-haired, dark-skinned girl said. "I've been having a great time and have met a lot of great people."

Kristen found out in third-grade, at age 8, that she was a person with diabetes. "I was pretty mad and upset about it," she recalled. "I often wondered why it was me that got this disease. I didn't think it was very fair for me to have diabetes when others didn't get it."

After all, who could blame her? Research has shown that diabetes can strike any one, at any time, without warning. It knows no age limits, gender limits or racial limits, though it may be possible that blacks may suffer disproportionately from the disease.

Kristen injects herself twice a day with insulin on a sliding scale. Having lived with this disease for some time has given her a new perspective on life.

"The one thing I can say to people who have come down with diabetes is to stay in control of yourself and do whatever it takes to keep it under control," she said. "You can live with diabetes; all you have to do is keep plugging away and do what you have to do."

Kristen aspires to teach middle school in the future. "I've wanted to teach for some time," she said. "I think I can be a very good teacher."

Mariko Powell
Age 14, Simpsonville, S.C.
Has attended Camp Adam Fisher for seven years:

Unlike many children who have to go off foods and drinks with sugar almost cold turkey when they come down with diabetes, Mariko Powell has never had any idea what a Coca-Cola Classic, for instance, tastes like.

That's because she came down with diabetes at the age of 9 months.

"I remember being stuck with needles and everything," Powell said. She's a dark-haired, slightly freckle-faced girl on the edge of becoming a beautiful woman who hasn't lost her sense of humor (a T-shirt she wore when she was being interviewed had a display of what we think are the charter members of the Ex-Boyfriend Hall of Shame). "But I really never knew how serious my disease was until I was 8 or 9, when I was wondering why my friends could have these things and I couldn't.

"When my mom told me about my disease and told me exactly what it was about, I was very upset. I knew that I would always want to have a candy bar or a Coke."

Of course, having had diabetes so long had a few benefits. "The things I do for my disease are like a second nature for me," Mariko said. "It's not like I suddenly got it a couple of years ago; it's something I've always lived with, so I never had to make the adjustment to having diabetes after having had things all my life. I've never been able to have things with sugar in them."

And that long experience helped when a friend of hers suddenly came down with diabetes. "My best friend came down with it, and I was able to help her through the adjustment period because I have always had it," she said. "It was very hard for her when she found out she had diabetes, but we were able to talk about it and get through it all right."

Brian Ashmore
Age 17, North Augusta, S.C.
Has attended Camp Adam Fisher for two years:

Like most people who get diabetes at Brian's age, the popular image of having to eat a boring diet and having to have an ultra-regimented lifestyle wasn't the most appealing thing for him.

One look at Brian shows he's not exactly boring: a modern-day hair style with braids, a goatee and a great sense of sports fashion: a Florida Marlins baseball-style shirt from Starter.

I guess the 1994 baseball strike hasn't dictated his fashion sense.

"I was 10 years old when I came down with diabetes," Brian recalled, "and the first thing I thought of was having to eat health foods and live a boring life. I mean, I couldn't even believe I had come down with diabetes.

"Needless to say, I soon learned that wasn't exactly true."

Brian follows a routine in which he checks his sugar level three times a day and gives himself two injections a day. "I was pretty scared about having to shoot myself with insulin, but one day, I just decided to do it. I'm all right with it now; it's just something I do as part of my daily routine," he said.

His friends also watch out for him whenever they go out. "Whenever we're playing something, they try to take it easy on me and make sure I'm all right," Brian said. "They always carry food for me and know what to watch for if I get into trouble."

Brian's future plans include hopefully getting into radio or television as a disc jockey or even an anchor on ESPN's popular *SportsCenter* sports news program.

"You just have to watch yourself and take care of yourself," he said."

Marcus and Martinez Scotland
Both age 15, Anderson, S.C.
Martinez has attended Camp Adam Fisher for five years,
Marcus for three years:

Diabetes isn't an unusual disease in the Scotland household.

Besides the twins, their father and sister also have the disease;

all four of them have to give themselves injections to survive.

"It's not really that hard," Marcus said. "It's something you

have to live with. It runs in my family, so seeing everyone have

to inject themselves isn't a big deal."

The disease hasn't stopped them from being active, normal

teen-agers. At the talent show during the 1995 Camp Adam Fisher

session, the two did a hip-hop dance routine that had the crowd

on their feet screaming for more.

"Being at camp is an unique experience, but it's also a lot of

fun," Marcus said. "We've met a lot of great people from all over

the state, and the experiences we've had are experiences we won't

forget."

Being with these special kids, even for a day, would be a real inspiration for anyone who would visit Camp Adam Fisher. There is so much that a person can learn about diabetes from these children.

In a previous chapter, one of the camp's directors wished that everyone in South Carolina could spend a day at Camp Adam Fisher to see just how remarkable these children are.

It is my wish, as well.

Camp Adam Fisher is something every other state should copy; the kids with diabetes in the United States would love the Palmetto State and the camp's organizers for it.

CHAPTER 23

It's Not Just in the Blood

===============

Diabetes just isn't about having to control your blood sugar levels. It's also having to worry about the complications that can come with it.

Here's a case in point: When we were putting out that special section in Rocky Mount, N.C., (which was a 72-hour marathon session for all of us), I developed eye trouble. An ulcer had somehow developed in my right eye, causing my vision to become blurred and causing me great pain.

I remember going home at about 3 o'clock in the morning and waking up the next morning with one eye closed and the other eye nearly closed sympathetically. I had not yet been diagnosed as a person with diabetes, but I'm willing to bet today that my blood sugar level was running at least at the 500-600 level.

If that ulcer had been just one millimeter higher, I would

have lost my right eye entirely. Thankfully, Dr. Bill Sheppard in Rocky Mount monitored my situation very carefully over the weekend, and within a week or so, my eyes were back to normal. It was at that time that I began to notice the weight loss and went to the doctor; the rest, as they say, is history.

But there's no doubt I nearly lost my eye because of diabetes; just look at the symptoms I was having.

Now, here's something to think about if you're a person with diabetes:

On the average, regardless if you are a Type I or Type II diabetic, chances are you've probably lost 5-10 years off your lifespan *unless* you keep the disease under tight control, watch your diet, exercise and take your medication daily.

The complications of diabetes from cardiovascular disease, kidney disease, blindness and neuropathy can be endless if you don't do what you are supposed to do.

Dr. John Colwell said that those with Type II diabetes risk cardiovascular disease probably threefold as compared to the norm. People with Type I diabetes, on the other hand, have a lot of potential renal (kidney) and eye problems. The key, Colwell believes, is using the Glucometers and keeping things under as tight control as possible.

Dr. Rob Lindemann adds that amputations don't have to take place; the same goes for kidney failure and other types of problems diabetes can bring on. "Between 60-80 percent of the complications of diabetes could be prevented if people would simply do what they are supposed to do.

"Seven to eight million people have Type II diabetes and don't even know it. Many Type II patients have it for six months, if not a year, before they learn they have diabetes."

The most important thing to remember: If you exhibit any of the symptoms of diabetes, you should immediately consult a physician. If you are diagnosed, the key is to keep it under control and listen to your doctor.

Your eyesight, your limbs, your kidneys are very precious to you. If you ignore what's going on, it's a sure bet you'll wind up paying for it in the long run.

However, proper treatment of diabetes can be more of a help than a hindrance to a person's lifestyle. A 10-year study conducted by the National Institutes of Health and sponsored by the National Institute of Diabetes and Digestive and Kidney Disease released in 1993 revealed that intensive treatment which keeps blood-sugar levels as close to normal as possible definitely reduces possible kidney, eye and nerve damage that diabetes can cause.

The study, called the Diabetes Control and Complications Trial, compared two treatment methods in 1,441 patients with insulin-dependent diabetes at 29 clinics in the United States and Canada. In the study, patients on intensive treatment used three or four insulin injections or an insulin pump to keep glucose levels as normal as possible. The patients adjusted their doses according to food intake, exercise and tests performed by a finger prick four times a day.

In the comparison group, conventional treatments that prevented symptoms were followed. This included one or two injections a day, daily blood sugar testing and a standard nutrition and exercise program.

Dr. Phillip Gorden, director of the National Institute of Diabetes and Digestive and Kidney Diseases, said, "Intensive treatment improves blood glucose control, delays the onset of diabetic eye disease and slows the progression of eye disease that has already started."

The study said intensive treatment reduced diabetic eye disease, or retinopathy, by 74 percent, while kidney disease, or nephropathy, was reduced by 35-56 percent and nerve disease, or neuropathy, by 60 percent.

Not bad for a disease that costs Americans $7.26 *billion* a year to treat and costs the American economy some $40 *billion* annually in health-care costs and lost work time, mostly because of blindness, kidney failure, nerve damage, amputations and heart disease.

CHAPTER 24

Feet, Don't Fail Me Now!

Dr. David Stellwagen knows what it's like to see someone lose a limb to diabetes.

As a podiatrist who specializes in treatment of foot problems and disorders because of diabetes, he's had to amputate the feet and legs of many persons with diabetes.

It's never an easy thing for him to do.

"I do a lot of amputations, but I hate it," Stellwagen, whose practice is based in Seneca, S.C., says. "It is absolutely an awful thing to have to do to someone, but sometimes, it's a choice of either seeing the patient die or seeing the patient lose a limb.

"If it comes down to that, I'll choose a person's life every time."

It is not a decision Stellwagen – or any podiatrist – takes lightly. Comparing diabetics to non-diabetics, the diabetic patient is 17 times more likely to develop gangrene, which can lead to the amputation of feet and other limbs.

The foot problems associated with diabetes account for more hospital stays than any other reason every year. According to research conducted and a medical article written by Drs. George P. Kozak and John L. Bowbotham, 14 percent of people with diabetes are hospitalized each year, averaging six weeks per stay.

Foot problems caused by diabetes – considering the ever-escalating health-care costs in the United States – can get to be pretty expensive, even for those who have full health insurance.

And these problems are something Stellwagen would like to prevent.

Stellwagen got into the practice of podiatry because of his mother. She had diabetes and had to see a foot doctor on a regular basis because of the complications diabetes can produce.

"It was hard for her to be disciplined in her diet and to keep an exercise regimen going," Stellwagen said. "Diabetes and foot problems are almost synonymous with each other, and without a doubt, it's a major public health problem.

"She really took poor care of her feet and herself, and she had to go to see podiatrists on a regular basis. Talking to her doctor (who was in Sacramento, Calif., where Stellwagen lived at the time) got me interested in podiatry."

Many people believe the foot problems caused by diabetes come from poor circulation. Surprisingly, that's not necessarily the case.

"It's not a case of poor circulation, although that can become a factor," Stellwagen said. "More than 20 percent of all diabetics have excellent circulation in their feet. What causes the foot problems is the progressive degeneration of the sensory nerves in the foot, the nerves that let people know what they can feel in the foot area.

"A person can injure a foot and never even know it, or they might not cut a toenail properly and wind up with an infection and never know it. Diabetes is a multiple-system disease, anyway, and the immune system is greatly weakened. Cuts and bruises don't heal particularly well, and patients are very prone to infections."

Statistics show that 60,000 lower-extremity (foot and lower leg) amputations are performed each year on those with diabetes. Foot problems are the No. 1 cause of hospitalizations among all people with diabetes. The most common foot problems that diabetics have are blisters, corns and calluses caused by poorly fitted shoes, warts on the foot, fissures, fungal infections, ingrown toenails and a problem that can arise when toenails aren't trimmed properly.

Stellwagen's mother became one of those statistics.

"My mother had a callus on her foot that suddenly became ulcerated," Stellwagen recalled. "The infection spread and later invaded the bone area, and she was in the hospital three or four times because of it. She never allowed the doctors to amputate her foot to relieve the problem.

"The doctors at Kaiser Hospital in Sacramento would debride the ulcer and treat her for the problems it was causing. I tried to help her as much as I could, but it wasn't easy to see her suffering."

Amputation of a limb because of diabetic conditions is never an easy decision, nor is it a particularly cheap procedure.

"The cost of a six-week hospital stay for a diabetic amputation can range between $10,000-16,000, and when you include rehabilitation, lost time from work and other factors, it can cost our economy some $300 million a year," Stellwagen said. "I personally try to help my patients all that I can, and I encourage them to get professional treatment for their problems. It's an awfully tough problem, though; I can tell you that from experience."

How can a person with diabetes prevent the potential problems that loss of feeling in their feet can cause?

"Every person with diabetes should seek professional foot care at all times," Stellwagen said. "Whenever I examine a person with diabetes, I check for possible infections, I check for potential trouble, I trim their toenails if they need to be trimmed and I always advise my patients to wear good-fitting shoes. That way, they can avoid foot problems.

"All a person with diabetes has to do is let a podiatrist help them take care of their feet, and it's likely they'll never face an amputation."

Chapter 25

New Waves of Treatment

Diabetes educators are becoming more and more common these days. In fact, there are about 8,000 registered diabetes educators in the United States, Canada and other countries. Through their efforts, they take a lot of pressure off physicians because they are able to help new diabetes patients become educated about the do's and don'ts of this disease. They can also change a patient's medication (with a doctor's permission) and help his or her family members learn more about the disease.

They do a great deal to help patients learn survival skills and help draw a picture of what could happen if sugar levels exceed 200 for patients.

Cindy Floyd of Seneca, S.C., is just such an educator. She receives several calls from people with diabetes each day seeking advice or counseling about diabetes and what to do to treat it.

Unlike some other educators, Floyd's advice is free; she is employed by Oconee Memorial Hospital in Seneca as a patient educator. "You get people of all walks of life and all intellectual levels here," Floyd said. "You have to get to their level and make sure they really understand what they need to do.

"No one can control diabetes without understanding the disease. You have to understand the basics of what goes on inside the body. If you understand why things are a certain way, you can avoid doing the wrong things."

Floyd has a simple way of looking at diabetes for her patients. "The first thing I get patients to understand is when you put gas in a car, you get a certain amount of mileage," she said. "Food, once digested, is the body's fuel that goes into the bloodstream (the gas line) on its way to the cells (the engine). If there is a break in your fuel line, the fuel never reaches the engine.

"For the person with diabetes, a break in the fuel line is when there is a lack of insulin, which allows the food (fuel) to enter the cell. Insulin is like a key. Sugar in the bloodstream knocks at the door of a cell. Sugar can only enter in if insulin is there to unlock the doors. When insulin is not there, the fuel never gets to the engine.

"Your fuel tank is full (your blood sugar is high), but you

are still 'out of gas' if it can't get into the engine (the cell)."

Floyd is a member of the American Association of Diabetes Educators, an organization "dedicated to advancing the role of the diabetes educator and improving the quality of diabetes education and care," according to the AADE's literature.

The goals of the organization include:

- To advance the role of the Diabetes Educator as the primary provider of diabetes education;
- To advance diabetes education as integral to the care of people with diabetes;
- To promote access to quality diabetes education for all people with diabetes;
- To develop and maintain an organizational structure responsive to members' input; and;
- To promote standards and guidelines for quality diabetes education.

Floyd knows she has helped a lot of people since becoming an educator, but she also realizes many people with diabetes don't realize she exists.

"I'm free," she said. "I have so much information I can provide people. As an educator, I have to make time to schedule patients in.

I check their medication, look at their diaries (used to track blood-sugar counts, food intake and insulin injections), vital signs and when they are in the hospital, sit at their bedsides and tell them that I understand what they are going through. I just feel I have worlds of information that is sometimes not being used."

Dr. Rob Lindemann says diabetes educators offer exceptional help to patients.

"Certified diabetes educators and nutritionists are up-to-date on the latest developments in diabetes," said Lindemann. "Education is extremely important, and it shows statistically, the more educated a person with diabetes is, the better the patient will do."

Floyd understands the stresses doctors are up against in seeing so many patients each day.

"A physician doesn't have time to teach in his office," said Floyd. "We can take more time with the patient. But the patient has to take on the role of caring for him or herself."

Surprisingly, Floyd never had any intention of becoming a diabetes educator. She had been a nurse at Oconee Memorial Hospital, rising to become third-shift supervisor of nurses. She had a wonderful husband, Haynie, and was pregnant with their first child when she began to have headaches, along with blurred vision.

Floyd knew it could be serious and had several CAT scans done. The results of the tests were shocking.

Floyd had a brain tumor behind her left eye, attached to her optic nerve – while she was pregnant.

During the pregnancy, nothing could be done to keep the tumor from going out of control and spreading.

The baby, named Marlie, was born in March 1984, and by January 1985, Cindy had gone to Allegheny Memorial Hospital in Pittsburgh to undergo treatment. Because of the location of the tumor, surgeons were unable to remove it, but were able to perform a biopsy, which showed the tumor to be benign. A plate was later inserted in her skull, and radiation treatments began.

While in the hospital, some terrible things happened to Cindy. An uncaring nurse ripped off a tube, taking some skin with it, and the wrong tests were done on Cindy several times.

Then, by July 1986, after having her second daughter, Holly, a MRI scan revealed the tumor was growing, forcing Cindy to travel to Greenville (S.C.) Memorial Hospital to do battle with the tumor during the Christmas holidays.

Radiation treatments and the problems with the tumor have cost Floyd her sight in her left eye; she also has only 20 percent upper right-side peripheral vision in her right eye. Straight ahead, Floyd has 20/15 vision in the eye, but because of the problems, she was forced to give up her job as graveyard-shift nursing supervisor.

"It was absolutely devastating," Floyd said. "I had always wanted to help people this way, but the hospital was very supportive during my problems and helped me in any way they could."

When a position for a patient educator became open, she applied for it and was hired, a decision she has not regretted. She became certified as a diabetes educator in 1991.

Her eyesight problems have given her a greater understanding of what patients with diabetes go through when it comes to similar complications. Her own vision problems make her much quicker to notice similar symptoms in people with diabetes and quick to offer solutions on how to avoid the complications.

Cindy has helped me immensely in my battle against diabetes by giving advice and answering any and all of my questions about the disease. I have learned so much from her, as much as I have learned from almost all the physicians I have come in contact with since I came down with the disease in February 1994.

"I would certainly encourage other people to take advantage of the advice from any certified diabetes educator out there," Floyd said. "We have the latest information about diabetes and treatments for the disease."

CHAPTER 26

If You Don't Stop It, You'll Go Blind

Diabetes can lead to many complications, as already documented so vividly earlier in this book.

Amputations are one of the most visible and dreadful complications of this disease. But diabetes can also lead to something perhaps even more serious than the loss of a limb – the loss of eyesight.

After all, a limb can be replaced by a prosthetic device. Once gone, eyesight can never be restored.

Canadian-born Dr. Joseph Parisi has seen what the ravages of diabetes can do to people with healthy, normal eyesight.

"The big thing is, people who need to be screened for possible problems because of diabetes aren't even aware of the fact that their vision can be damaged, even destroyed, by this disease," Parisi said. "Many times, people only become aware of the problems after it is too late to do anything about it."

There are things people with diabetes need to be aware of when it comes to their vision. They are at much higher risk for contracting cataracts (spots on the lens of the eye that cause vision to become cloudy and eventually blurred) and glaucoma (a disease of the eye in which internal pressure from the eye's fluid builds up to the point where vision is impaired). Both diseases of the eye can be corrected rather easily.

The most serious problem most persons with diabetes must worry about is a condition called diabetic retinopathy, a disease in which changes in the blood vessels that surround the retina takes place. (The retina is the area at the back of the eye which takes "pictures" of what is being seen and relays the message to the brain.)

Sometimes, blood vessels in the retina swell and eventually spring leaks. Other times, new vessels form on the retina's surface, which can cause loss of vision, a detached retina or even blindness. The horrible thing about these conditions is that there is usually no warning about what is going on until it may be too late.

"Once someone gets an advanced case of retinopathy, there isn't much we can do about it," Parisi said. "The vessels in the retina are very fine ones, and under pressure, like they are with a person with diabetes, they can burst, start to leak or cause other problems to a person's vision.

"Usually, these retinal walls are pretty watertight, but with a person with diabetes, the walls are broken down. The vessels suddenly begin to leak, and by the time I see the patient, there's a major problem."

Blindness can result from the condition, especially for those with diabetes who are dependent on insulin.

"That's why people with diabetes need to set up and follow a regular schedule of eye exams," Parisi said. "People with diabetes especially need to be seen on a regular basis because of what could happen.

"I treat many diabetics, and if we can catch problems early, we can recommend a course of therapy that can help them retain their eyesight. We can never fully repair damage already done, and we can never eliminate the risk of blindness, but with regular screenings and treatment, we can certainly make the risk very manageable."

Not only can early detection and treatment save a person's eyesight, it can also save people money in the long run.

"There was a study done by Johns Hopkins University in Baltimore about the social and economic cost of diabetics who go blind," Parisi said. "It can cost people a lot of money.

"Given the need to get health care costs under control in this country, people are talking about trying preventive medicine. That, and the maintenance needed for diabetic eyes, can really help a patient."

The American Diabetes Association recommends persons with diabetes get an eye exam at least once a year, and when problems are found, to get on a treatment program as soon as possible to prevent damage and loss of eyesight.

"If someone has to have surgery, it won't necessarily improve their vision," Parisi said. "But we usually retain some sight, and having some eyesight is better than blindness."

CHAPTER 27

The ADA: From Professional to Personal

Persons with diabetes don't have to suffer this disease alone.

Thanks to two major organizations, persons with diabetes can have access to the latest information on their disease, on how to cope with daily problems, how to diet, how to exercise and even find out about support groups available in their areas.

The American Diabetes Association (ADA) is the oldest of the two major organizations set up to fight diabetes and its complications. It offers memberships to the general public, to persons with diabetes and to professionals who are active in health care, education and/or involved in diabetes research. It has been in the forefront of many breakthroughs in the treatment of the disease.

The American Diabetes Association was founded in 1940 by 26 physicians as a professional society dedicated to finding better ways to treat people with diabetes. It led the fight to recognize those with diabetes as normal, everyday people by ongoing educational programs and efforts to fight higher life insurance premiums and on-the-job discrimination.

The ADA published, in conjunction with the American Dietetic Association and the diabetes branch of the U.S. Public Health Service, the first food exchange and meal-planning guides for diabetics in 1950. These were updated in 1979 and again in 1986 and 1995.

In 1953, the ADA helped produce the first mass screening programs to detect diabetes and helped introduce the first test strips for blood glucose levels in 1964, the biggest advance in diabetes care since the introduction of insulin in January 1922.

The ADA, realizing that diabetes had become a major problem in American health, reorganized itself in 1969 as a national voluntary health organization. It immediately announced plans to support more research into, advocacy for and education about diabetes to the public at large, which was still largely ignorant of the disease and its consequences.

The ADA is currently based in Alexandria, Va., and has affiliates and chapters in more than 800 communities in all 50 states and the District of Columbia. The organization was formed "to prevent and cure diabetes and to improve the lives of all people affected by diabetes," according to ADA literature.

The ADA has affiliate headquarters in major cities in each of the states to coordinate individual local and state fund-raising and educational activities. The organization has more than 1 million volunteers and a membership roll of 265,000 patients and their families, plus a professional membership of thousands of physicians, scientists, nurses, dietitians, pharmacists, social workers and educators.

Many chapters and affiliates offer all sorts of activities for those with diabetes, their families and friends, including educational classes, youth programs, counseling and support groups, advocacy services (including lobbyists in all 50 state capitals and in Washington for federal matters) and referral services. ADA services and research extends to 70 countries internationally.

The ADA publishes a monthly magazine, *Diabetes Forecast*, which offers feature articles on people with diabetes and tips to help the person with diabetes enjoy a rewarding lifestyle. It offers cookbooks and meal guides to help those with diabetes control their disease and books, brochures and pamphlets for both persons with and without diabetes to help them understand the disease. The ADA also publishes several professional journals covering every aspect of the diabetic world and the status of research on the disease.

Educational programs include the American Diabetes Alert, held annually to alert the public about the dangers of diabetes and to urge those who may be at risk from the disease to obtain medical testing, and National Diabetes Month, in which activities are geared toward prevention of the disease for those who may be at risk.

For professionals, the ADA also offers educational programs designed with them in mind and places emphasis on the improvement of care of people with this disease. Programs include scientific sessions held annually, an annual post-graduate course for diabetes clinicians, several other seminars and symposiums, medical care guidelines and recommendations based on the latest information and an accreditation program for diabetes patient education.

Thanks to the ADA's efforts, $90 million has been invested nationwide into diabetes research. Some recent advances in this research have resulted in more precise and accurate ways to identify persons at risk for diabetes and its complications and explore potential treatments to prevent the onset of diabetes; improved techniques for islet cell transportation; laser therapy techniques to prevent blindness brought on by diabetes; a better understanding of the role good nutrition plays in diabetic treatment, as well as a better understanding of the psycho-social factors that affect such treatment; a better understanding of how maintaining tight blood glucose levels can benefit patients; and movement toward finding possible genetic causes of diabetes.

As part of its fund-raising efforts, the ADA sponsors several national events each year, including The Neighborhood Check for Diabetes, in which neighborhoods are canvassed with information about diabetes; Walktoberfest, an annual event each October where thousands of people take a walk to raise funds for diabetes research; and the Tour de Cure, a bicycle touring event for cyclists to help raise funds for diabetes research.

The ADA has also been active in the Hispanic and African-American communities with specialized programs designed to get diabetes information to these people who may not have the resources to learn about and cope with the disease. A telephone service, known as DIAL, provides diabetes information at the toll-free number (800) DIABETES to both persons with and without diabetes.

For 55 years, the ADA has been a leader in the United States on helping persons with diabetes live normal lives. That mission continues even stronger today and will not stop until a cure is found.

For more information on the American Diabetes Association, write to 1660 Duke Street, Alexandria, Va., 22314, or call toll-free (800) 232-3472.

CHAPTER 28

JDF CURE

Super Bowl XX, played at the Louisiana Superdome in New Orleans Jan. 26, 1986, brought national attention to the Juvenile Diabetes Association.

Jim McMahon, the Chicago Bears quarterback whose use of various promotional headbands had already been thoroughly discussed, used one emblazoned with the words "JDF CURE" before the game. The NBC commentators explained the significance of the saying to the vast TV audience.

After all, it's a wonder what some 80-100 million viewers nationwide, tuned in for one of the biggest sporting events around, can do for an organization.

The JDF, based in New York, has helped many people with diabetes over the years with its research and educational efforts to find a cure for the disease. It was started by a group of parents whose children suffered from diabetes and who wanted them to live better, happier and healthier lives than what was thought possible at the time.

Ever since the organization was founded, it has had one simple goal: The complete elimination of, and a cure for, diabetes in people of all ages and all walks of life. It has chapters and affiliates in every state and in the District of Columbia, coordinating activities and efforts in each of its state affiliates for people with diabetes.

Thanks to JDF-sponsored research, early detection of diabetes has become possible. Work is currently progressing, in addition, on agents to prevent the disease and possible genetic links to diabetes.

In recent years, JDF-funded research has led to two major breakthroughs for those with diabetes. The development of an external pump for insulin distribution has helped many people avoid the dreaded daily injections. An internal pump has also been developed in South America; it is currently in use in Brazil and is awaiting approval for use in the United States.

In 1990, the JDF stepped up efforts to find a cure for diabetes, declaring this decade as "The Decade for the Cure" of this disease. Increased fund-raising and educational efforts were launched, reaching millions of people throughout North America. Funding for research into the disease also picked up steam in this all-out effort.

In 1994-95, the JDF awarded $19.5 million for diabetes research as part of its "Decade for the Cure" campaign. Included in those grants was money for research in 11 states, four Canadian provinces and 15 other nations on four continents. Since the first grants were awarded in 1974, the JDF has supplied a total of $156 million for research into diabetes worldwide.

The JDF also supplies people with and without diabetes with information and educational pamphlets and booklets about the disease and seeks to play a role in continued state and government support into research into diabetes, its causes and a possible cure for the disease. Its best-known spokesperson is actress Mary Tyler Moore. A number of other celebrities have also taken up the cause for diabetes research, including Alan Thicke, Gloria Loring, John Ratzenberger and Susan Ruttan.

For more information on the Juvenile Diabetes Foundation, write to 432 Park Avenue South, New York, N.Y., 10016-8013 or call toll-free (800) JDF-CURE.

CHAPTER 29

Racing, Cycling and Walking for a Cure

═══════════

When it comes to raising funds for diabetes, there are as many ideas as there are those with diabetes.

In the South, NASCAR stock-car racing is a near-obsession, and two stock-car racing-related events have proven to be major fund-raisers for diabetes-related research and education in recent years.

But racing isn't the only way to raise money for the American Diabetes Association, the Juvenile Diabetes Foundation and other diabetes-related outlets. In this chapter, we'll take a look at some of the ways money is raised for the fight for a cure throughout the nation.

THE MARK COLLIE CELEBRITY RACE
NASHVILLE, TENN.

Country music fans know about Mark Collie from his many hit records and songs he's written for many other Nashville recording artists, songs such as *Hard Lovin' Woman, Even the Man in the Moon is Crying, Born To Love You, Shame Shame Shame Shame* and *She's Never Coming Back* and for stars such as Randy Travis, Marty Stuart, Aaron Tippin, Martina McBride and Collin Raye.

What fans may not necessarily know is that Collie himself is a person with diabetes.

"I have had insulin-dependent diabetes for the past 17 years," Collie has said, "and I know first-hand how much more must be accomplished in education and research (into the disease). I realize and understand the complications that affect children, as well as adults, who survive daily the injections, special diets and fitness regimens that help to cope with diabetes."

Collie was first diagnosed as a person with diabetes when he was 17 years old, back in 1977. But he didn't let his disease stop him from moving to Nashville from his hometown of

Waynesboro, Tenn., to try to make it in Music City USA.

To this day, Collie continues to be an outspoken advocate of public education about, and research into a cure for, diabetes.

As many fans know (and others are learning quickly), country music and NASCAR stock-car racing have always gone together like many other great combinations in the Southeast (the late Marty Robbins, in fact, drove in several Winston Cup races, including the Daytona 500, before his 1982 death, and many other current country performers have written songs about stock-car racing), so perhaps that was the impetus for Collie putting together a race in 1994 at Nashville Motor Speedway to benefit the American Diabetes Association and the Juvenile Diabetes Foundation and also to establish a research grant at Vanderbilt University in Nashville in honor of Larrie London, a well-known Nashville session player who died from complications from diabetes.

The race, known as the Mark Collie Celebrity Race for Diabetes Cure, presented by HealthSouth (a regional medical care company) saw some 10,000 music and racing fans crowd into the NMS facility on Oct. 13, 1994. An associated auction and VIP event helped the two-day happening raise nearly $200,000 for the Mark Collie Foundation for the battle against diabetes –

despite stormy weather that swept through central Tennessee.

The event drew both country music stars and legendary NASCAR drivers such as Kix Brooks and Ronnie Dunn (Brooks and Dunn), T. Graham Brown, Lorianne Crook and Charlie Chase of The Nashville Network, Rodney Crowell, Joe Diffie, John Hiatt, Faith Hill, Greg Holland, The Mavericks (Trisha Yearwood's backup band), Tim McGraw, Delbert McClinton, David Lee Murphy, Joe Bonsall and Richard Sterban of The Oak Ridge Boys, Stella Parton, Doug Phelps (Brother Phelps), Marty Roe (Diamond Rio), Nashville radio personalities Karl Shannon and Bubba Skynyrd, Lisa Stewart, Doug Stone, Steve Wariner, Joy Lynn White, Lari White, Mike Alexander, Bobby and Donnie Allison, Buddy Baker, Dick Brooks, Richard Childress, Red Farmer, Elliott Forbes-Robinson, Harry Gant and Coo Coo Marlin (father of two-time Daytona 500 winner Sterling Marlin).

All of them drove NASCAR Legends cars, 5/8-scale cars with a Yamaha motorcycle engine built to resemble the cars raced during NASCAR's pioneering days in the early 1950s.

The race's grand marshal was, and still is, the living legend and symbol of NASCAR – The King himself, Richard Petty, something Collie was very proud of. "I am especially honored that Richard Petty served as grand marshal," he said.

Speed wasn't that much of a factor during the evening, but the wet conditions did lead to some slipping and sliding on the quarter-mile NMS track. "A lot of folks were spinning, having a tough time keeping it straight," Roe, the eventual winner, told *Country Weekly* magazine. "Joe Diffie was rough on me; I don't know where he learned that driving technique. He bumped me a little bit, but I just went ahead and blew him away."

"It's like driving on ice out there," Diffie told the magazine. "The cars look like they're going real slow, but when you're in there, it's like a blur."

Wariner himself gained new respect for the drivers in NASCAR's elite Winston Cup series after he climbed out of his car. "I have a lot more respect for those NASCAR guys after I've tried it myself," he said. "It's another world."

By the time the event was over, though, few cared exactly what had taken place; the bottom line was that plenty of money was raised to find a cure for a disease that can strike anyone, anytime and anywhere – and everyone had fun at the same time.

THE CALE YARBOROUGH 500
GREENVILLE, S.C.

Cale Yarborough is another one of those living legends of NASCAR who has given freely of himself to help many causes throughout the Southeast.

But the three-time Daytona 500 winner and Winston Cup champion in 1976, 1977 and 1978 (even though he now has the pressure of running his own Winston Cup team and several other businesses near the Grand Strand area of South Carolina, near Myrtle Beach and Darlington) has not gotten more satisfaction and happiness out of the causes he has supported than the Cale Yarborough 500, a diabetes fund-raiser held in Greenville, S.C., one of the major cities in South Carolina's Upstate region.

In it, regional businesses make a donation to the American Diabetes Association's South Carolina affiliate to enable one of their employees to drive small-scale Winston Cup replica cars on a Greenville street course for fun, the honor of their firms – and for people with diabetes throughout the Palmetto State.

"The ADA office in Columbia contacted me a couple of years ago and asked me if I would be interested in doing this,"

Yarborough said from his Florence, S.C., car dealership office. "We went over the particulars of the idea, and I thought it was a very good one. I told them I would be honored to help them out.

"Even though my schedule is a very busy one, I'm always glad to give whatever time I can to help causes like this one."

Like many people who are involved in diabetes-related causes, Yarborough had heard of the disease, but never really thought about it until it hit close to home.

"I had a best friend who came down with diabetes," Yarborough said, "and I soon learned there is no doubt that anyone, anywhere, can get this disease, from the big-name businessman to the average person on the street.

"Seeing him go through what he has really brought home the reality of diabetes to me, and since then, I've been very dedicated to diabetes causes. I want to do all I can to help find a cure for diabetes and to educate the public about diabetes."

The 500, in fact, is a smart idea, Yarborough believes, thanks to the ever-growing popularity of NASCAR nationwide and the fact that the roots of NASCAR run deep in the Southeast.

"Whoever came up with this had a great idea," Yarborough said. "It not only creates interest in diabetes research and funding, it also gives families a chance to have a great time together and all the participants a chance to have some fun, maybe live out a few racing fantasies.

"It's definitely the most rewarding cause I've ever been involved in. I've enjoyed every second of this event."

OTHER FUND-RAISING IDEAS

The ways to raise funds to battle diabetes are limited only by the imaginations of the people who want to stage the events. Money is always needed by organizations like the ADA and the JDF.

Says Robbie Butt, marketing director for the ADA's South Carolina affiliate: "Money fuels the fire for research and education. Unfortunately, not enough members of the American Diabetes Association contribute extra funds. The past year, we were so successful at promotion of the ADA that our demands outstripped our support.

"There are many ways we can raise money, through individual contributions, memorial contributions, corporate support and fundraisers themselves."

Walks, runs, kiss-a-pig contests (where companies in a

locality put up a candidate in a fund-raising drive; the winner gets to plant a big wet one on a pig, which represents the source of insulin for many with diabetes), golf tournaments and even sporting clay competitions have become popular in the Southeast to raise funds for diabetes.

If you have an idea for a fund-raiser, contact the national ADA or JDF organizations or your local or state affiliate offices. They are always willing to lend a hand for a new fund-raiser.

Much of the money that is raised from these events goes to educational efforts and printing costs for diabetes brochures and booklets to get the word about diabetes out to the general public.

CHAPTER 30

Mountains to the Sea

Wayne Terry and his wife, Kathy, have never feasted on turkey and all the trimmings with their two children, Teresa and Lee, on Thanksgiving Day.

Instead, for the past 15 years, the Seneca, S.C., couple have spent their Thanksgiving weekends participating in the Mountains to the Sea Run, a fund-raiser for the American Diabetes Association's South Carolina Affiliate.

The relay run begins every year on Thanksgiving morning at the Georgia state line above Long Creek, S.C., and finishes 346 miles later on Saturday morning at the Landmark Resort Hotel in Myrtle Beach, S.C.

The Terrys get teary-eyed when they talk of what it has meant to them to assist their good friends, Maurice and Marlene Poore and other members of the Oconee County Road Runners Club, in their fight to find a cure for diabetes.

"I think it is just a great thing when you can get 20 people of different walks of life and unite them for a run of this nature for a charity," said Wayne Terry. "It takes a lot of time, planning and a commitment each person makes to take three days to do this.

"But we've always decided we were going to do the run. We haven't been together with our kids on Thanksgiving weekend, like most families, but with all of those who take part in the Mountains to the Sea Run."

Robbie Butt and Kristin Epting, of the ADA's South Carolina office, proudly accepted a check for $20,000 after last year's run, which was the best ever. The annual run has raised more than $150,000 in its 15-year existence. The money has gone to help spread diabetes awareness and assist in research to find a cure.

The idea for the run was the outgrowth of a commitment of a small group of neighbors to Sherri Morrison, who was diagnosed with diabetes at age 9. Sherri was advised by her doctor to participate in some strenuous activity to burn off and control her excess blood sugar.

She chose to walk and run, and her father, Maurice Poore,

and their neighbors chose to participate with her on the quiet country roads around her home in the Ebenezer community near West Union.

The group of neighbors formed the Oconee Road Runners Club, which then decided they wanted to do something for a charity and, because of Sherri, chose diabetes for the run.

Joe Dowis, a Westminster, S.C., schoolteacher, came up with the idea to run to Myrtle Beach and do the long run as a club fund-raiser. The first run raised a total of $2,976.39 and took about 41 hours over a 310-mile course.

Kathy Terry remembers jogging through snowflakes when they started the first run.

"We were sore and whipped, but we got there," said Wayne Terry of the first run. "It took us 41 hours and 23 minutes."

The Oconee Road Runners had little support from law enforcement officials and other running clubs in the beginning, but that has now changed. The South Carolina Law Enforcement Officer's Association, South Carolina Sheriff's Association, Clemson University Track & Track Club, the Anderson Roadrunners, the Greenwood Running Club, the Columbia Running Club, the Marion Pacers Roadrunners Club and AWHFY all participate in the run every year.

Shoney's restaurants and Hardee's restaurants eventually started feeding the run's participants, but in the beginning, it was a pretty steady diet of cold-cut sandwiches for those taking part.

In 1985, the run started having police escorts. Before that, it was up to the Oconee Road Runners' van to be the escort. Showers were usually hard to find during the grueling trip, and few stores were open. One time, a South Carolina Highway Patrol officer pulled over the van and asked what they were doing.

"We scampered around to find a letter from the State Highway Patrol Department about what we were doing," said Maurice.

The run raised about $6,000 in 1985. Media publicity started to take off at this point, and the police became more involved.

In 1988, the run raised $10,000, and by 1991, $13,000 was raised. After years and years of making the trek to Myrtle Beach, the run was well established. Corporate sponsorship has increased every year and continues to escalate.

During the early years of the run, Maurice and Wayne recalled time after time when they had to climb out of the van and run five or six miles if someone who had already signed up failed to show. Somehow over the 15 years, they have always dug within their souls to complete each portion of the 300-plus mile challenge.

"Everyone has put forth so much effort," said Maurice. "Words aren't there to describe the feeling I have about these people doing this every year. They have reached back and done it so many times. There have been 15 years of everyone giving up Thanksgiving weekend."

Wayne and Maurice had to fight back tears when they were talking about the commitment it has taken each year to complete the run.

"You become like family when you do something like this every year," Maurice said.

Maurice's original hope was that the run would be duplicated in other states and, on Thanksgiving weekend across America, similar runs would take place. He said that hope has somewhat faded.

The Mountains to the Sea run is a perfect fund-raiser that can be put on anywhere. A similar run could be done river-to-river or even from one portion of a state to the next. This type of fund-raiser does take a lot of courage, commitment and planning, but then again, that's exactly what made America!

I take my hat off to the Terrys, Poores and all others in the

Oconee County Road Runners Club who for the past 15 years, have given up their Thanksgiving weekends to assist in the battle against diabetes.

"They have done it through thick and thin," said Butt. "Doing this for 15 years has taken just an unbelievable commitment."

The $150,000-plus dollars raised by these heroes from the small country roads in Oconee County, S.C., have done much to assist the ADA in its education and research process.

CHAPTER 31

The Diabetes Lobby

Fact: In 1989, $4 billion was spent on AIDS research in this country.

Fact: In the same year, $288 million was spent on diabetes research.

Fact: Since January 1986, there have been 267,479 deaths attributed to HIV/AIDS.

Fact: In 1990 alone, 162,567 people in the United States had diabetes or diabetes complications on their death certificates.

"I saw these figures about three years ago in Washington when the American Diabetes Association and International Diabetes Federation brought key executives together," said Dr. Rob Lindemann, who has been very outspoken about the proportion of funds devoted to AIDS research vs. diabetes research.

"Diabetes is a terrible disease, too, killing many more people than AIDS. Those in the AIDS lobby have done a good job of being politically correct and promoting their cause. We need to be more aggressive in going after federal funding and private dollars.

"I think we need to do a better job of publicly spreading the word. We should spend more money doing national TV advertising. The squeaky wheel, after all, gets the oil."

Often, people with diabetes seem to keep quiet. The diabetes lobby does appear to be getting stronger and more vocal, however, with much more awareness being spread by organizations like the ADA and Juvenile Diabetes Foundation.

"People seem embarrassed and don't want to talk about diabetes," said Lindemann. "We need to make more noise in trying to raise funding. Private industry gives away money to the American Heart Association and many other organizations. We should get more money from that source. The JDF does a good job of raising funds for research. We all need to be active and aggressive for the cause."

Lindemann cited an example of a California endocrinologist friend who doesn't even tell his patients he has diabetes.

"He's trying to be secretive, but so many of his patients would appreciate how he feels if he spoke to them personally about the disease," Lindemann said.

Steve Smith has done much lobbying in the state of South Carolina for diabetes. He agrees with Lindemann that diabetes research funding is very disproportionate, compared to AIDS.

"We need to increase the awareness level about diabetes in the coming years," Smith said. "I will personally be spending much of my time lobbying for diabetes until we find a cure."

Smith was a leading force in lobbying to obtain funding for the South Carolina Diabetes Initiative, created by the South Carolina General Assembly in July 1994. A Diabetes Initiative of South Carolina Board oversees the statewide program of education, surveillance, clinical research, and translation of diabetes treatment methods to serve the needs of South Carolina residents with the disease.

A total of $159,000 in statewide funding was obtained for the program. Hundreds of volunteers across South Carolina helped the initiative pass through the legislature. The grassroots work took place over a two-year period.

This type of state-funded program has made South Carolina a front-runner in education, surveillance, research and treatment methods. Other states are constantly inquiring about the program in hopes of enacting something similar in their part of the country.

Dr. John Colwell has been another major guiding force in helping to get the Diabetes Initiative passed.

"Dr. Colwell recommended we do a study to see the impact of diabetes in South Carolina," said Smith. "It is a dream come true for Dr. Colwell, who is internationally known. He is such a special person. He is the architect behind the Diabetes Initiative.

"Our research has found that diabetes and its complications fill one out of every seven hospital beds in South Carolina and cost patients an estimated $600 million in 1993."

Colwell is extremely proud of the Diabetes Initiative, which he worked on for several years.

"We worked on the program for several years," Colwell said. "We put together a survey in 1992-93 studying the scope in South Carolina and made a recommendation to the legislature on what to do.

"The study involved a national committee of representatives working on diabetes. The Department of Health and Environmental Control, the Governor's office and many others were represented on the 15-person committee, which met monthly to draft a report. The report was submitted during the 1993-94 fiscal year. It felt promising. It was submitted in January and carried over into session in 1994. In June 1994, we passed the Diabetes Initiative in South Carolina."

A Diabetes Center of Excellence has been established at the Medical University of South Carolina in Charleston. The center has made health professional education as its main priority. It is also responsible for conducting Diabetes Initiative board meetings and overseeing the flow of activities surrounding the Initiative, including fiscal responsibility.

A Surveillance Council works closely with DHEC and studies costs, mortality, morbidity, blindness, amputations and other health factors in which diabetes plays a role. Much of this information is obtained from hospital discharge and insurance data.

The program has been so successful that other states have inquired about setting up similar programs. Texas was one of the first states to conduct a program like the one in South Carolina, which includes public awareness of diabetes and an outreach program to at-risk families throughout the state.

Another interesting lobbying effort took place in Massachusetts with a diabetes "Day on the Hill" March 22, 1994, at the Massachusetts State House in Boston in conjunction with the ADA's annual American Diabetes Alert. The effort was organized by health agencies to raise awareness among state legislators about the seriousness of diabetes and its health-related care issues.

With widespread support, the Massachusetts Affiliate plans to make Day on the Hill an annual event to coincide with the American Diabetes Alert on the third Tuesday in March.

I can only encourage others to realize the importance of speaking out about diabetes and its effects. Without grassroots efforts like the ones in South Carolina, Massachusetts and Texas, we will not spread the word to the American public how serious diabetes and the complications surrounding the disease can be.

Without increased awareness, more will die each year from personal ignorance about the disease and poor treatment. We must continue to educate our physicians on the latest trends and ways to treat this illness.

Diabetes should be taken as seriously as other killer diseases like AIDS. This will only happen through our efforts in lobbying for the cause.

CHAPTER 32

What Does the Future Hold?

Like any disease, there are many questions about diabetes and what the future may hold for people who have it.

Questions still abound: What causes it? Why does it run in some families? Why do members of the black community get it in disproportional rates?

And, of course, the main question: Is there a cure in the future?

Actually, when you think about it, treatment for diabetes has come a very long way. Back in ancient Egyptian times, diabetes was treated by mixing ground dragon's blood from the Elephantine with flax and onions, then boiled in oil and honey and taken for four straight mornings.

Not the most tasty breakfast, to be sure.

Some 3,000 years later, research advances into both the cause and control of diabetes have done much to help the millions of people with diabetes out there in the United States and the world. In fact, since insulin was discovered by Canadian researchers Drs. Frederick Banting and Charles Best in the 1920s, people with diabetes have had more than a fighting chance to live happy, normal lives.

Dr. John Colwell sees a lot happening with the genetics of diabetes in the future. He also sees more advancements in ways to test blood sugar without having to stick one's fingers with needles several times a day.

"A lot is being learned about the genetics of diabetes," he said, "such as molecular identification and learning about kindrids."

Dr. Rob Lindemann sees many things happening in the future, possibly an implantable closed-loop insulin pump that would free many with diabetes from having to inject themselves, as well as further work in diabetes prevention trials, which helps spot markers in children who could be potential diabetics.

Lindemann also says there may be something one day that people with diabetes can be given to stop the immune-system breakdown process from happening. He also sees strong potential for pancreatic implants.

Dr. Bob Laird hopes to see more genetic manipulation so

we do not see diabetes anymore, while Dr. Frank Axson doesn't see the insulin pump as being the cure-all to the disease; it's a bit overwhelming, he says. But he, like Lindemann, sees pancreatic implants as the wave of the future.

The American Diabetes Association itself is continuing a study, co-sponsored by the National Institutes of Health, called the Diabetes Prevention Trial – Type I, or DPT-I. It is the first study of its type to determine whether Type I diabetes can be prevented through the administration of low doses of insulin to people at high risk for the disease. There is a strong possibility that such doses, as shown in the landmark 1993 Diabetes Control and Complications Trial, conducted by the National Institutes for Health, may not only hold off the disease, but prevent the most serious complications of diabetes, such as kidney damage, blindness and nerve damage that can lead to amputation of the extremities.

It is important to note that there is still a long road to travel before results of today's research becomes reality. But thanks to this research, the day may come when newspapers blare headlines about a cure for one of the most devastating diseases known to man.

On that day, all of us will rejoice.

CHAPTER 33

A Non-Diabetic Reacts

========

By BRENT FEENEY

I guess living with diabetes isn't the easiest thing in the world to do.

I've never had it myself, so I feel fortunate. But I do know someone who has diabetes.

He's my boss at work. He's the guy who came up with the idea for this book. He's the guy who has seen it grow to what has been, hopefully, a great guide to life for all of you readers out there.

More importantly, he's my best friend.

We've been through all sorts of things together, starting back in the summer of 1988 when he hired me as sports editor of *The Daily Standard* (later *The Standard•Democrat*) in Sikeston, Mo., right on top of the southeastern Missouri Bootheel region.

I had just graduated from Eastern Illinois University in Charleston, Ill., and, yes, Dan graduated from there, as well (he graduated from EIU in 1982, two years before I arrived on campus). Over the years, even with many disagreements, arguments and who knows what else we've been through, we've both stayed as loyal to each other as any two friends could be.

We were in Rocky Mount, N.C., back in February 1994 when everything broke loose. Dan hadn't been feeling well for some time, but at this particular time, we were in the middle of putting together a special newspaper section for the upcoming Rocky Mount Chamber of Commerce banquet. It was right in the middle of that year's Winter Olympics in Lillehammer, Norway, and we had been pulling some pretty grueling all-nighters to get this section together. (I remember drifting off to sleep a couple of times right in the middle of the sessions.)

I think it really started when Dan had trouble with his eyesight. He complained of very blurred vision and a burning sensation in his eyes. We all looked at him, and his eyes looked like they had gone 15 rounds with George Foreman.

We all decided that he had better get himself home and go to a doctor as soon as he could; we were concerned that he might have gotten a photographic chemical into his eyes, which would have caused some pretty serious problems.

I don't remember the exact date, but when I saw Dan after his visit to the doctor, I asked him what the verdict was.

"It's not good," he said to me. "I've got diabetes."

"WHAT?!?," I said to him.

"I've got diabetes. I'm sick. I've got a disease which is going to be with me the rest of my life."

Needless to say, I was shocked, devastated, stunned – insert your own descriptive word in this space.

Diabetes? I knew it was around; even knew about some famous people who had it. Being a big sports fan, I knew Catfish Hunter had diabetes. I knew Bobby Clarke had diabetes. Both of them had led teams to championships in their respective sports (Hunter in baseball, Clarke in hockey).

I knew it was a disease that could be controlled, and I knew people could lead successful, productive lives with it.

But my best friend? Someone I had nearly hated during the worst of times and had helped during some very difficult times and someone I had always considered one of the best friends I had ever had in my life?

NO WAY!

WAY!

At that moment, I didn't know what to do. I don't think I could do anything. I just sat in the chair, letting Dan's announcement sink in.

When Dan started his own paper, called *The Bridge*, he asked me to come join him that Thanksgiving. Having nowhere else to turn, and seeing the loyalty Dan was showing to me, I jumped at it.

It was tough. The paper was just a month old, and I wasn't making very much money. But we hung in there and seemed to have the corner turned.

That's when Dan's diabetes struck. The next few months were a horrible roller coaster ride; he'd work for a bit, go home to rest, come back, rest, etc., every day. It was tough.

Dan's physical appearance took a terrific beating. He had always prided himself on being in great shape, lifting weights, running and later swimming, to stay in shape. But as the diabetes took hold, it was obvious the pills he had been taking weren't working.

His weight dropped from the 190s to the low 140s. He would do situps at my apartment when he came to visit me, and I could see right through to his ribs. It was a horrible and sickening sight; I told him he was starting to look like a concentration camp survivor. He was ghastly pale, his hair was falling out and he generally looked as though a good stiff breeze might knock him down.

I was convinced he didn't have diabetes, but cancer or AIDS instead. I felt he wasn't telling me the truth because he didn't want me to worry about him.

I confronted him a few times, and he kept telling me he had diabetes. I finally believed him when I saw him test his blood sugar level and give himself a shot for the first time.

Boy, talk about stomach-wrenching! Hearing the needle break the skin was about as fun as seeing the average horror film these days.

Gradually, I saw Dan return to normal. These days, he's as healthy as he's ever been.

I'd hate to think what might have happened had he not gone on insulin or, worse, not been diagnosed as a someone with diabetes.

Every day, I'm learning more and more about diabetes, about the care and feeding of those with diabetes, about what he can have and what he can't have, about how regimented the life of a person with diabetes – simply by necessity – must be.

Because of Dan and some of the other people I've talked to for this book, I've learned so much about diabetes, its treatments and complications.

These people have been an inspiration for me. They have not let this horrible disease get them down; in fact, they have shown that they can conquer diabetes and show it who's boss, especially the kids I talked to at Camp Adam Fisher one warm Saturday in June 1995.

My wish is that you have learned something about diabetes through this effort and will take it more seriously. There are millions of people with diabetes in this nation alone; your mom, your dad, your wife or husband, your boyfriend or girlfriend, your best friend, your closest relative, even your sibling, may have diabetes.

It's more common than you think, but it's not a disease that puts you on your behind for the rest of your life.

Chapter 34

Some Conclusions

Writing a book is not an easy task.

For me, the endeavor has taken almost all my free time during 1995.

I have learned so much about diabetes through interviewing people in the medical profession, talking to organizations like the ADA and JDF and talking to people who have struggled and, in all cases, learned to survive with this illness.

The past year and a half hasn't been easy for me. I've learned a lot about myself by becoming a person with diabetes.

There have been many hard times. I have over and over wondered why I was selected as one of such a small fraction of the population that has take insulin each day just to live.

I've learned I had to keep getting up each day and facing the reality I cannot do things as before. I have to test my blood sugar four times a day, whether I like it or not.

At the moment, I am seeing Dr. Paul Davidson, a diabetes specialist in Atlanta and taking four insulin injections each day. I have to constantly watch my diet and avoid certain types of foods.

The illness humbled me a great deal. Before, I seemed to have it all, but in reality, I didn't. Having it all is much more than being singularly focused on a career.

Thanks to this illness, I have been found many times on my knees praying to the Lord for help and guidance. I am thankful for waking up each morning.

I no longer have my wife and family with me, but I know when I do get a second chance, I will be different. My priorities will be God, family and career, distinctly in that order.

It will take a special person to be married to me. The emotional ups and downs with diabetes are difficult, but I know if someone really loves you, they will be able to cope. The spouse will also have to help watch your diet, encourage, assist with shots and always be on guard for hypoglycemia.

I feel fortunate to have been able to write this book. Of course, I don't have all the answers and do not consider myself a medical expert. The book has been a means of cleansing my aches, reexamining (or redefining) my hopes and coping with this entry in, as Carroll Gambrell calls it, "a different world."

I am a common, everyday person who hopes to spread the word about a disease which can cause serious complications or be a killer for those who do not play by the rules.

But I am not the only person who should get credit for this book. During the research and writing of this book, I had some help from a person you met in chapter 33, a person who is my best buddy – Brent Feeney.

There have been times when I don't know if I would have made it or not if he wasn't around. I don't think that this book would have ever come off if he hadn't been around to help me.

Thanks, Brent.

I also want to thank the numerous people who helped me edit and put this book together. Most of all, I want to thank my family and friends for not giving up on me. Once you go through things like losing a business and becoming a person with diabetes, one really appreciates the family and friends who are loyal to you through the good and bad times.

If you are recently diagnosed or have been a person with diabetes for a long period of time, you have nothing to be ashamed of. Unfortunately, inside you was a genetic makeup which enabled you to have diabetes.

One of the problems is people with diabetes have not spoken up through the years. Because of that, diabetes has not gotten the federal or state funding it has needed, as compared to diseases like AIDS. I'm not saying finding a cure for AIDS isn't important; I just think our priorities should be more balanced than they are now.

I'm looking forward to seeing improvements in the insulin pump, insulin, treatment methods and improved technology for people with diabetes in the future.

I hope and pray someday, there is a cure. I'm thankful for the life I still have ahead. I am bound and determined to make the best of whatever is ahead, no matter what I must face. I am also determined to be outspoken about the disease and will talk to anyone, at any time and in any place, in trying to help them understand what it is like to be a person with diabetes.

Don't be afraid to cry. Don't be afraid to talk the talk and walk the walk about the disease, or as I did, get on your knees to pray to your Savior.

If you play by the rules in this new, and somewhat complicated, world, diabetes can be an interesting way of life.

Most of all, I want to give thanks to all the medical efforts over the last 75 years that has helped all of us live full and productive lives.

Through their efforts, and the gutsy determination that lives in us all, we've proven to the world that, without a doubt, diabetes does *not* have to be a death sentence.

Want to order some more copies?

To order additional copies of
Life To The Fullest,
just send a check or money order to:

Dan Brannan Publications
P.O. Box 1708
Seneca, SC   29679

Name:_____

Address:_____

City, State, ZIP Code:_____

The book is $15.95 per copy, plus $3 postage and handling for the first copy
Please enclose 50 cents per additional copy requested.
S.C. residents add 5 percent sales tax

FOR QUANTITY DISCOUNTS, WRITE:

Marketing Director
Dan Brannan Publications
P.O. Box 1708
Seneca, SC   29679

Tear here

Want to order some more copies?

To order additional copies of
Life To The Fullest,
just send a check or money order to:

Dan Brannan Publications
P.O. Box 1708
Seneca, SC   29679

Name:_____

Address:_____

City, State, ZIP Code:_____

The book is $15.95 per copy, plus $3 postage and handling for the first copy
Please enclose 50 cents per additional copy requested.
S.C. residents add 5 percent sales tax

FOR QUANTITY DISCOUNTS, WRITE:

Marketing Director
Dan Brannan Publications
P.O. Box 1708
Seneca, SC   29679

Tear here

Want to order some more copies?

To order additional copies of
Life To The Fullest,
just send a check or money order to:

Dan Brannan Publications
P.O. Box 1708
Seneca, SC 29679

Name:_____

Address:_____

City, State, ZIP Code:_____

The book is $15.95 per copy, plus $3 postage and
handling for the first copy
Please enclose 50 cents per additional copy
requested.
S.C. residents add 5 percent sales tax

FOR QUANTITY DISCOUNTS, WRITE:

Marketing Director
Dan Brannan Publications
P.O. Box 1708
Seneca, SC   29679

Tear here